MECHANICAL NECK PAIN
Perspectives in Functional Anatomy

JAMES A. PORTERFIELD, P.T., M.A., L.A.T.

President and Owner, Rehabilitation and Health Center, Crystal Clinic,
 Akron, Ohio
Adjunct Faculty, Cleveland State University and The Ohio State University

CARL DeROSA, P.T., Ph.D.

Professor and Chairman, Physical Therapy Program, Northern Arizona University,
 Flagstaff, Arizona

W.B. SAUNDERS COMPANY
A Division of Harcourt Brace & Company
PHILADELPHIA, LONDON, TORONTO, MONTREAL, SYDNEY, TOKYO

W.B. SAUNDERS COMPANY
A Division of Harcourt Brace & Company

The Curtis Center
Independence Square West
Philadelphia, PA 19106

Library of Congress Cataloging-in-Publication Data

Porterfield, James A.

Mechanical neck pain: perspectives in functional anatomy / James A. Porterfield, Carl DeRosa.—1st ed.

    p.   cm.

ISBN 0–7216–6640–X

1. Neck pain—Pathophysiology.   2. Human mechanics.   I. DeRosa, Carl.   II. Title.

[DNLM: 1. Neck—physiology.   2. Cervical Vertebrae—physiology.   3. Pain. WE 708 P849m   1995]

RC936.P66   1995

617.5′3—dc20

DNLM/DLC   94–12257

MECHANICAL NECK PAIN: Perspectives in Functional Anatomy   ISBN 0–7216–6640–X

Printed in the United States of America.

Last digit is the print number: 9   8   7   6   5   4   3   2

To Sara, Christopher, and Patrick DeRosa,
and Alison and Jeffrey Porterfield.
The joy and love you bring to our lives
help keep our efforts in focus.

ACKNOWLEDGMENTS

We are indebted to the following individuals for their assistance and encouragement throughout this endeavor: Laura Berton, L.A.T.C., Chris Baker, M.S., L.A.T.C., Catherine Blount, and Dave Bacha, M.D., Ira Fritz, Ph.D., Vert Mooney, M.D., Richard Borden, P.T., Ph.D., and Don Greenbaum, Ph.D. Finally, a very special thanks to Tina Cauller for her exceptional work and creative suggestions and her willingness to listen, discuss, and ultimately translate ideas into pictures.

PREFACE

The human neck is the most mobile region of the spinal column, being in nearly continuous motion throughout the day and even as we sleep. It is remarkable that through an area allowing such exceptional movement pass some of the most delicate and vital structures for life such as the spinal cord, esophagus, trachea, and carotid and vertebral arteries. Precise, reflexive motor control of the head and neck is provided via an intricate and uniquely sophisticated neuromuscular machinery.

The purpose of this text is to discuss in detail the structure and function of the cervical spine and to develop a practical clinical model by which the clinician can effectively assess and treat painful disorders. If improperly managed, disorders of the neck can become disabling because of their influence on every activity from our gestures and resting postures to our ability to perform work.

As in its companion text, *Mechanical Low Back Pain: Perspectives in Functional Anatomy,* a foundation in the neurosciences, articulations, and associated musculature of the cervical spine provides the framework for evaluation and treatment, emphasizing prompt restoration of function and education for self-management. A comprehensive understanding of the functional anatomy of the cervical spine affords the clinician the basis for keeping patients active. At the same time the clinician must recognize that physiological loading capabilities of tissues are adversely affected by injury, age, and the degenerative processes.

The authors advocate that the prognosis for most activity-related neck disorders is quite favorable, as it is in low back problems. Successful treatment outcomes depend upon patient education, which places the patient in an active role during the treatment process. Such an approach minimizes the potential for neck pain to become a disability. The authors hope that the information presented in this textbook provides practical tools for clinicians as they strive to be successful in dealing with mechanical disorders of the cervical spine

JAMES A. PORTERFIELD, PT, MA, LAT
CARL DeROSA, PT, PhD

CONTENTS

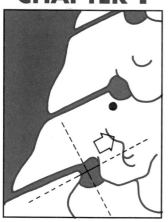

CHAPTER 1

PRINCIPLES OF MECHANICAL NECK DISORDERS

THE NECK PAIN PROBLEM

The epidemiology of neck disorders is understood to a much lesser degree than that of low back disorders. Investigation of the cervical spine has lagged behind that of the lumbar spine for the most part, and an analysis of the prevalence and incidence of neck disorders is no exception.

As with the low back, several factors hinder a comprehensive study of neck disorders. One is a lack of agreement on diagnostic classification. Epidemiological studies often fail to clearly differentiate neck pain from pain in the upper extremity, or the two regions are combined for analysis.[1] The lack of a standardized diagnostic classification system has hampered the generation of outcome studies because cervical spine syndromes, lacking clear definition and criteria, cannot be compared. In Chapter 5, a diagnostic classification system is suggested to enable better communication among clinicians dealing with neck disorders and, more important, to initiate the use of a common terminology that will promote the development of meaningful outcome studies.

Another factor is the lack of consensus regarding the treatment of neck disorders. Deyo has described various treatments for low back disorders that appear to be equally effective but that vary widely in cost.[7] There is no indication that the situation is different for neck disorders. Treatments include pain modulation interventions, such as electrical stimulation and topical modalities; manual and mechanical interventions, such as manipulation, joint mobilization, soft tissue work and traction; and various forms of neuromuscular training, such as posture instruction and resistive exercises. Consistency in treatment is increasingly recognized as essential because it has the potential to help control the escalation of costs for spinal disorders and to allow for comparison between outcome studies.

Other considerations that compound an accurate assessment of the epidemiology of neck disorders are the influences of legal, psychological, and social factors. Gay and Abbott noted more than 30 years ago that the institution of litigation often stimulates a self-perpetuating cycle of pain and anxiety in patients suffering from whiplash injury of the neck.[13] Many believe that this holds true today as well. Norris and Watt, however, demonstrated that litigation in neck disorders is more dependent on the severity of injury than on neurotic tendencies.[32] Determining the severity of neck injuries and the prognosis for recovery is no simple task, as evidenced by Gotten's study

1

demonstrating that a wide divergence of opinion exists among surgeons when they are called on to give expert testimony in legal disputes.[14]

Macnab reviewed 145 patients 2 or more years after settlement of litigation and found that 121 were still having neck symptoms. In another review of 266 cases, he found that 45 per cent continued to have symptoms after settlement of claims.[29] Macnab notes that with such a large number of patients still having complaints after settlement of litigation, it is unreasonable to dismiss these patients as hysterical or neurotic.

PREVALENCE OF NECK DISORDERS

Several attempts have been made to study the prevalence of neck problems. Prevalence is a measure of the number of people in a given population who have the syndrome or disease at a particular time. Several studies provide insight as to the prevalence of neck problems. Hult noted that the prevalence of neck pain in industrial and forest workers ranged from 35 to 71 per cent.[20] Takala and colleagues suggested that the prevalence of neck pain in a middle-aged population was 18 per cent in women and 16 per cent in men.[40] About 10 per cent of the population will develop neck pain, with or without referral of pain into the upper extremities, during any given month.[2]

Dvorak and co-workers' extensive review of 11,423 patients with neck pain, conducted over a 3-year period, analyzed the mechanism of injury and suggested that 87.5 per cent of these cases were soft tissue injuries, 53 per cent resulted from motor vehicle accidents, and 45 per cent were caused by other types of injuries, mainly falls and sporting accidents.[8]

INCIDENCE OF NECK DISORDERS

The analysis of the incidence of a problem provides epidemiological information that differs from studies of prevalence. Incidence refers to the rate at which individuals develop a syndrome or disease over a specific time. Disc disorders provide a good example of studies directed toward an analysis of incidence. Although the incidence of lumbar disc herniations exceeds that of cervical disc herniations, several studies have analyzed the incidence of disc pathology related to the cervical spine. Kondo and associates noted a cervical disc herniation incidence of 5.5 per 100,000 for men and women, with those in the 45- to 54-year age group being most often affected.[23] The disc level most commonly involved is C5-6, followed by the C4-5 and C6-7 levels.

Kelsey and colleagues analyzed groups of people who were diagnosed as having cervical intervertebral disc disorders over a 2-year period. They noted that people in their 40s were more likely to be affected by such disorders than those in other age groups.[22] Moreover, the results of their study suggested that several factors are associated with cervical intervertebral disc disorders. They are frequent lifting, diving from a board, and cigarette smoking. Less significant than these but still showing an association with cervical disc disorders is the time spent operating vibrating equipment and driving motor vehicles.[22]

Social factors also need to be considered when analyzing the prevalence or incidence of cervical spine disorders and cervical spine associated upper-extremity disorders. A good example of the influence of societal factors is in the review of the epidemiology of repetitive strain injuries. The current epidemic of repetitive strain injuries and cumulative stress injuries is well known.[18, 21, 28] There is not clear evidence, however, that the problem is solely ergonomic or biomechanical. The Telecom study from Australia suggested that there is little relation between the escalation of repetitive strain complaints of cervical and shoulder origin and changes in technology, ergonomics, or workplace factors.[18] Instead, repetitive strain injuries were more related to social influences, job dissatisfaction, and the society's legitimation of this type of injury. The epidemic of two problems related to cervical spine and upper-quarter disorders—carpal tunnel syndrome and temporomandibular joint syndrome—might have the same phenomena as contributing factors.

Clearly, the knowledge base for cervical spine disorders is much more limited than that for lumbar spine disorders. Because low back disorders have had the greatest economic impact on society, they have logically been the focus of the most intense study. However, patients with neck pain alone or neck pain with associated upper-extremity problems continue to represent a significant proportion of cases of spinal disorders.

On closer inspection, there are marked similarities between the etiology, pathogenesis, and prognosis of low back pain and the etiology, pathogenesis, and prognosis of neck pain, just as there are similarities between the anatomy and mechanics of the lumbar spine and the anatomy and mechanics of the cervical spine. The aggravating factors and the resolution of mechanical neck pain are similar to those of low back pain. In most patients, acute neck pain resolves in about 1 month with a rapid, uncomplicated course.[2] A much smaller number of patients develop chronic pain syndrome despite conservative or surgical care. The latter group is responsible for the greatest proportion of the medical costs, and therefore, an understanding of the psychological factors that contribute to chronic pain syndrome is indispensable for appropriate management.

Despite such an array of complicating factors, increased attention is being paid to the economics, epidemiology, assessment, and management of neck pain. The problem often is debilitating because neck postures and movements are important components of social expression. An understanding of the nature of the problem allows the clinician to more efficiently utilize the history and physical evaluation to provide appropriate treatment and patient education.

THE CERVICAL SPINE AS A COMPONENT OF THE UPPER QUARTER

Epidemiological studies of neck pain suggest that the cervical spine may be only one component of neck pain complaints. Structures related to the upper extremity and head often are involved with the painful syndrome, and an examination of these structures reveals alteration in function. Thus, it is necessary not only to study the detail of the cervical spine itself, but also to recognize how it influences and is influenced by surrounding structures.

The development of the cervical spine has resulted in an exceptional degree of mobility. Forces attenuated through the cervical spine are largely due to the weight of the head and upper trunk and the forces of muscle contraction. Because of the interplay between the occiput, mandible, cervical spine, upper thoracic spine, shoulder girdle, and arm, this complete region is referred to as the upper quarter.

The uniqueness of the cervical spine and the interplay between different tissues of the upper quarter are exemplified by noting selected regions of specialized anatomy and their resulting contributions to function.

1. The vertebral column supports the weight of the occiput, and the ligaments and muscles must be able to counter the moment of inertia of the head (Fig. 1–1). Thus, a large weight (the head) is placed on disproportionately smaller bones (the cervical vertebrae), which demands

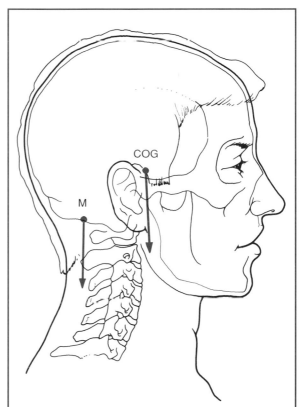

Figure 1–1. Sagittal view of the head and neck with the location of the center of gravity of the occiput. The center of gravity is countered by the contractile state of the extensor muscles of the occiput and cervical spine. COG, center of gravity.

that an intricate interplay exist between ligaments and the neuromuscular system to counterbalance the weight of the head.

2. Several organ systems are directly related to the upper quarter, and therefore, the tissues of the neck must contain and provide a degree of protection to vital structures. These structures include the vertebral artery, internal jugular vein, sympathetic chain of the autonomic nervous system, and components of organ systems, such as respiratory and digestive tissues. These structures must be taken into consideration during assessment of patients with cervical spine disorders.

3. The cervical vertebrae not only house the spinal cord and nerve roots, but the upper cervical vertebrae are directly related to the lower regions of the brain stem (Fig. 1–2). Stability of the region is crucially important, yet unique adapta-

tions have been made to provide a great deal of mobility.

4. It is difficult to completely assess the cervical spine without also assessing the shoulder girdle. The bones of the shoulder girdle provide anchors for muscles that attach to the occiput and cervical vertebrae, and the shoulder girdle must be effectively anchored if muscles connecting the cervical spine to the scapula are to exert an effect. In addition, referred and radicular pain patterns require that tissues of the shoulder girdle be closely examined.

5. There is a wealth of reflex connections between various elements of the cervical spine and the special senses such as hearing, sight, and vestibular function. Disturbances of the receptors, the effectors, or component of the reflex connections result in clinical signs such as dysequilibrium and visual disturbances and often are a component of neck disorders.

A more detailed description of these and other aspects of the region's functional anatomy is provided in subsequent chapters.

A variety of painful syndromes occur as a result of injury or age-related changes of the tissues of the upper quarter. Even though the cervical spine is not subject to the degree of load that the lumbar spine or other weight-bearing joints typically encounter, it is a common source of pain. Compounding the clinical picture is the observation that the experience of pain in the cervical spine or related regions of the upper quarter can stem not only from injury or degeneration of the involved tissues but from psychological and emotional distress as well.

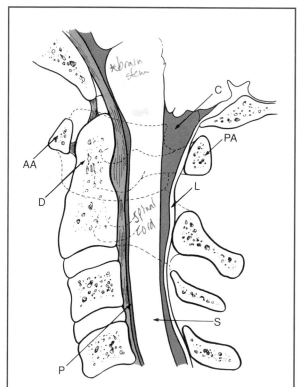

Figure 1–2. Sagittal view of the cervical spine demonstrating the relation of the brain stem and spinal cord to the vertebrae. AA, anterior arch of atlas (cut); C, cisterna magna; D, dens; L, ligamentum flavum; PA, posterior arch of the atlas; P, posterior longitudinal ligament; S, spinal cord.

THE PATHOMECHANICAL BASIS OF ASSESSMENT AND TREATMENT

A confounding question raised after evaluation of any area of the spine is whether the exact tissue at fault can be identified. It is difficult to precisely identify the anatomical source of pain with most spinal disorders. The assessment process can yield a diagnostic conclusion that is largely influenced by examiner bias rather than by the actual symptoms and signs encountered. In addition, it often is unreasonable to assume that one isolated tissue is at fault because the mechanism of injury or the changes that occur with the degenerative process affect multiple tissues rather than one tissue or structure in isolation.

As an alternative to attempting to identify the precise anatomical tissue at fault with neck pain, an assessment process for mechanical neck disorders should focus on the pathomechanics of injury and the reproduction of pain with the application of various stresses to the tissues of the cervical spine and upper quarter. An important feature of the evaluation process for mechanical neck disorders is analyzing the forces applied to the upper quarter during the physical examination, such as compression, tension, and shear, and noting the effect such forces have in reproducing familiar signs or symptoms. The ability to reproduce familiar signs or symptoms through the application of forces during the physical examination and an analysis of the forces that resulted in tissue injury as gleaned from the history allow the clinician to arrive at a pathomechanical rather than an anatomical diagnosis.

Such an approach does not preclude one from attempting to isolate pain to precise structures but instead provides a meaningful data base from which the clinician can develop treatment strategies designed to minimize those forces that excessively load injured tissues. More important, the patient can be better instructed in regard to occupational or daily living activities that potentially place the same type of stresses through the injured region. Such a strategy becomes extremely important when educating the patient in self-management strategies for the mechanical neck problem. This approach depends on an understanding of the functional anatomy of the cervical spine and the upper quarter.

Even without identification of the precise tissue that is injured, methods of managing spinal disorders have more similarities than dissimilarities and are comparable in intended outcome. In Chapter 6, the objectives of treatment are discussed and the different techniques required to meet these objectives are reviewed. Many of the techniques have the same short-term intended outcomes. It is the long-term result, however, that is the most important measure of the success of the treatment process.

As mentioned above, one primary intent of the management process for mechanical neck pain is to optimize the opportunities for the patient to become involved in his or her treatment process. Self-management strategies are important in the treatment of spinal disorders, especially as cost-containment measures become an even more crucial issue. Education for self-management strategies minimizes the likelihood that the patient will become dependent on the clinician for the mechanical neck problem. Care for spinal disorders including the neck is rapidly changing from a passive approach to a more active one, especially since we understand that the natural history of symptom resolution is quite favorable. Clinicians need to realistically determine whether the purpose of treatment is to make the patient feel better or function better. More important, a focus on improvement of function minimizes the prospect of mechanical neck pain progressing to chronic pain syndrome.

Self-management and restoration of function are the primary goals in the management of mechanical neck pain. Because the only rational approach for treatment of the injured musculoskeletal tissues is a gradual, progressive, active exercise program that guides the repair process of injured tissues through the controlled application of stresses, an understanding of the basic tissues pertinent to the cervical spine is essential.

RESPONSE OF TISSUES TO STRESS

One common denominator among musculoskeletal tissues is that they must be subjected to nondestructive forces to maintain an optimal state of health. Tissues related to the upper quarter are no different. Figure 1–3 shows the theoretical physiological loading capacity of musculoskeletal tissues. The area under the curve identifies the regions in which tissues of the musculoskeletal system are subject to loads that are excessive or loads that are so minimal that the tissue is no longer adequately stressed. Both scenarios result in tissue breakdown, either through injury or as a result of the catabolic effects of inactivity.

The graph also depicts an optimal loading zone that would be unique and different for all tissues. This zone represents the physiological loading capacity of the tissues when subjected to such forces as compression, shear, and tension.

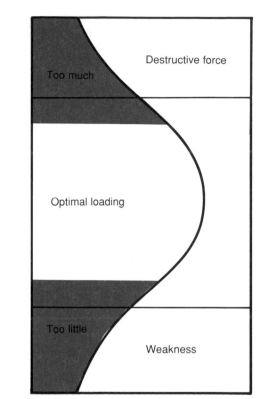

Figure 1–3. Optimal loading zone of musculoskeletal tissues.

Maintaining tissue loading within this region of the curve optimizes the capacity to sustain tissue health.

The boundaries of the optimal loading zone can be altered by several factors (Fig. 1–4). One is age. Several important changes occur with the aging process that affect the tissues' ability to attenuate stresses. Aging results in alterations in the concentration as well as the composition of proteoglycans. Changes such as a decrease in the concentration of chondroitin sulfate and the resultant increase in the keratan sulfate–chondroitin sulfate ratio occur.[15] In addition, there is an increase in both collagen and collagen-proteoglycan binding.[17] The combination of these factors decreases the availability of binding sites for water. Thus, the tissue becomes less hydrous and, subsequently, less resilient. The loss of resilience lowers the tissue's physiological loading capacity.

Aging leads to an increase in the density and

stability of collagen, primarily caused by cross-linking of the fibers.[38] As a result, there is an alteration in the stress-strain curve for connective tissues (Fig. 1–5). It is important to note that aging alters the steepness of the stress-strain curve, implying that the connective tissue is more vulnerable to progressive breakage of individual collagen fibers and frank rupture.

The extensibility of connective tissue is also altered with age. Elastin, which is 15 times more extensible than collagen, confers elasticity to the tissues.[38] With aging, the elastic tissue frays and the individual fibers become fragmented. Along with this change in elastin, there is a decrease in tissue water content and an increase in the viscosity of ground substance. As a consequence, the elasticity of tissues decreases.

Proteoglycans play a significant role in the

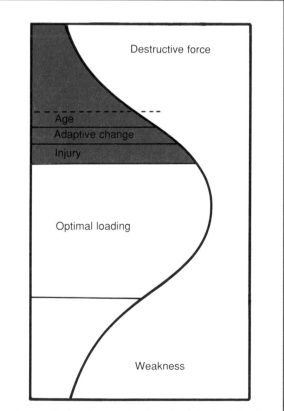

Figure 1–4. Change in the physiological loading capacity of tissues as a result of age, injury, and adaptive changes to the musculoskeletal structures.

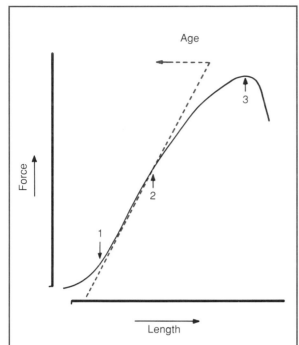

Figure 1–5. Influence of applied force on connective tissue length (tendon). Age increases the steepness of the force-length relation. Up to point 1, the fibers are lengthened. Between points 1 and 2, the elastic range of the fibers is reached. Beyond point 2, there is rupture of the individual fibers. At point 3, frank rupture of the connective tissue occurs. Aging increases the slope of the force-length relation.

function of connective tissue structures such as ligaments, joint capsules, tendons, and cartilage. Two of the key proteoglycans are hyaluronic acid and chondroitin sulfate. Hyaluronic acid is an especially viscous lubricant that allows elastic fibers, collagen fibers, and muscle fibers to slide over one another with minimal friction.[38] Chondroitin sulfate acts more as the bonding agent of the ground substance, which serves to stabilize the connective tissue structures. With aging, there is a decrease in the proteoglycan content and polymerization capabilities. As a result, the stability of connective tissue structures such as cartilage decreases.[38]

Through these mechanisms, age alters the shock absorption and shock attenuation capacity of the musculoskeletal system. As a result, the

limits before destructive loading occurs are lowered.

The second factor that decreases the force-attenuating capability of the musculoskeletal system is injury. The acceleration injury of the neck serves as an excellent example of the influence of injury on the future load-bearing capacity of the tissues. Severy and co-workers estimated that even in a relatively slow-speed, rear-impact motor vehicle accident (13 km/h or 8 mph), the head undergoes a 5g acceleration in less than 0.5 seconds.[37] This results in the physiological range of motion of the neck being greatly exceeded with resultant damage to ligaments, capsules, and muscles. The potential sites of tissue damage with this typical acceleration injury are listed in Table 1–1. Tearing and hemorrhaging of the longus colli, longus capitis, sternocleidomastoid, and scalene muscles frequently occur.[26] Cartilaginous damage is also common.

Tissue repaired as a result of injury such as that which might occur in the acceleration injury described above is different than normal, uninjured tissue. The injured tissue does not have the same force-attenuating capacity or the same viscoelastic qualities as the tissue it has replaced. As a consequence, it becomes subject to the injury-reinjury process. In oversimplified terms, injured tissue that has been repaired becomes the weak link in the musculoskeletal system. For example, injured ligaments do not regain their original tensile strength, and the range of recovery is only 50 to 70 per cent.[44] This is especially relevant to cervical spine acceleration injuries resulting in injury to the anterior and posterior longitudinal ligaments. As a result of such damage, a loss of cervical spine static stability might be expected.

Table 1–1. Potential Sites of Tissue Damage in Acceleration Injury

Anterior longitudinal ligament
Intervertebral disc herniation
Separation at bone-disc interface
Spinous process fracture
Muscle strain or rupture
Apophyseal joint sprain or fracture
Esophageal hemorrhage
Temporomandibular joint disruption
Vertebral artery ischemia
Sympathetic chain disorder

Experimental studies of muscle laceration reveal that muscle fragments heal primarily by dense connective tissue scar and that muscles lacerated near the midbelly recover about 50 per cent of their ability to produce tension and shorten about 80 per cent of their normal amount.[12] Repaired muscle is also more fatigable than normal muscle.[9] One might deduce from these studies that significant injury to the anterior neck muscles, such as the sternocleidomastoid or longus colli and capiti, as a result of the acceleration injury alters their function.

Such experimental data regarding ligamentous and muscle tissue underscore the fact that tissues that have been substantially injured, especially as a result of excessive application of force, no longer have the same physiological loading capacity as in the preinjury state. If this understanding is applied to the acceleration injury of the cervical spine, it influences management strategies. Certainly one goal is to restore function to as great a degree as possible, but more important, the patient and the clinician must recognize that some loss of function is inevitable with significant injury. Teaching the patient self-management strategies to maintain loading within the new capacities of tissue tolerance is essential.

The final factor that decreases the force-attenuating capacity of the musculoskeletal system is adaptive change of the tissues. Although the body has extraordinary compliance and is continually responding to stresses placed on it, changes in function become readily apparent when unyielding stresses such as prolonged postures and general inactivity ensue.

Posture influences many aspects of the musculoskeletal system and deserves special mention with a discussion of neck pain. More than is often realized, the nervous system is the major determinant of posture because of the barrage of sensory information from muscle spindles, tendon organs, and receptors related to joints and ligaments.[4] Posture is also markedly influenced by injury and psychological factors.[10] Posture becomes especially important to consider because the forces generated into and through the skeletal structures are attenuated by the precisely controlled coordinated actions of the neuromuscular system, which ultimately accomplishes the intended action. Adaptive postural changes strongly influence kinetic and static musculoskeletal functions.

One of the most common postures seen in patients complaining of mechanical neck pain is the rounded-shoulders, forward-head posture. This posture often is accompanied by weakened abdominal muscles and adaptive shortening of the anterior hip tissues. The relation between the weakened abdominal wall and the rounded-shoulders posture is further discussed in Chapter 5. The rounded-shoulder, forward-head posture features adaptive changes to the cervical lordotic curve; decreased occiput-atlas mobility from shortened posterior suboccipital tissues; shortening of anterior neck muscles, such as the scalenes and sternocleidomastoid; excessive tensile stress to the posterior spinal muscles, such as the levator scapulae and scapular retractors; altered scapular position; an internally rotated humerus; a decrease in the costoclavicular space through which the neurovascular elements related to the subclavian artery and brachial plexus course; and often a change in temporomandibular joint mechanics. Such widespread changes markedly affect the kinetic and static functions of the head, neck, thoracic spine, and shoulder girdle and alter the capacity of the tissues related to the upper quarter to properly attenuate forces.

These three factors—age, injury, and adaptive change—decrease the load-bearing and force-transference capacity of the musculoskeletal system. Forces generated into the tissues that exceed the upper-level capacity result in tissue damage, triggering the response of pain caused by mechanical or chemical activation of the nociceptive system. The role of the clinician is to assist the patient in maintaining an active, healthy lifestyle within the optimal loading zone so that excessive forces are not generated into an injured area. Interruption of the pain-spasm-pain cycle and patient education are primary goals in the treatment of mechanical neck disorders.

FUNCTION OF THE SPECIALIZED CONNECTIVE TISSUES

For the purposes of this text, the specialized connective tissues refer to bone, articular cartilage, and noncontractile connective tissues of the cervical spine, such as the intervertebral disc, supporting ligaments, and joint capsules. The specialized connective tissues, especially the bones and intervertebral disc, attenuate and transfer the forces of gravity and movement. The contribution of the neuromuscular system, by comparison, is to provide the "motors" that generate forces into and through these specialized connective tissues.

Bone

Two patterns are evident in the bones of the cervical spine, and each uniquely contributes to the attenuation of the forces of gravity and movement (the bony anatomy of the cervical spine is discussed in detail in Chapter 4). The first pattern, represented in cortical bone, consists of densely packed compact bone that provides great strength and rigidity to the skeletal system. The second pattern is cancellous bone, which provides a trabecular system of struts formed as a result of stresses imparted to the bone. One of the unique features of bone is its ability to alter its shape in response to stresses placed on it. *wolf's law*

The subchondral bone plate is the specific area of bone immediately below the calcific plate of the articular cartilage matrix of the synovial joint. The health of the subchondral bone plate ultimately depends on the load-bearing capacity and force-attenuating capabilities of the articular cartilage.

The bones of the upper quarter take many shapes and forms. The various articulations within the neck (upper cervical and lower cervical spine) provide a structure that confers exceptional mobility yet meets the demands of counteracting the weight of the head and offering a rigid lever system for muscle attachments.

Articular Cartilage

The articular pillars of the inferior and superior articulating processes are covered with articular cartilage. Articular cartilage is composed of collagen in a ground substance consisting of large mucopolysaccharides. Cartilage is unique in that it not only attenuates but also redistributes forces as they converge into the synovial joint. The structure of articular cartilage is shown in Figure 1–6.

The microscopic view of articular cartilage reveals an irregular and pitted surface (Fig. 1–7). These small indentations enhance the boundary lubrication function of cartilage because synovial fluid resides in the spaces between the two cartilage surfaces. Such an arrangement allows an exceptionally low coefficient of friction to exist between the cartilaginous surfaces (Table 1–2).

The articular cartilage is loaded in compression by the effect of gravity and the force of muscle contraction. With compression, fluid is expelled from the articular cartilage. With de-

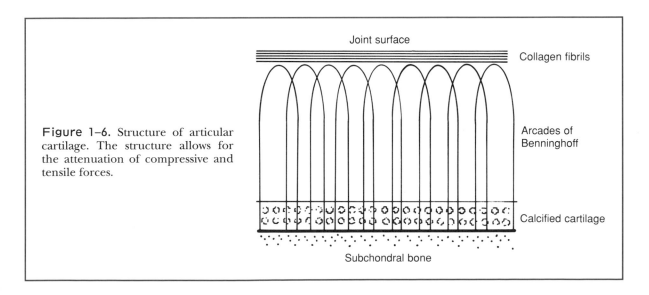

Figure 1–6. Structure of articular cartilage. The structure allows for the attenuation of compressive and tensile forces.

Joint surface

Collagen fibrils

Arcades of Benninghoff

Calcified cartilage

Subchondral bone

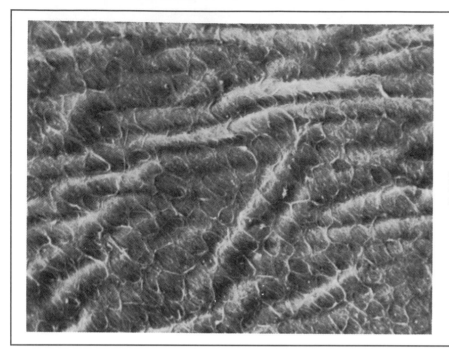

Figure 1–7. Pitted surface of the articular cartilage allows for the pooling of synovial fluid.

compression, fluid seeps back into the cartilage. This cyclic activity of compression and decompression maintains the health of the articular cartilage. Compression that cannot be unloaded diminishes the capacity for joint fluid and associated nutrients to seep back into articular cartilage. This accelerates the degeneration process.

An example of continuous, unyielding compression of the cartilage between the cervical articular facets is the forward-head posture (Fig. 1–8). Because the facet planes are obliquely oriented, the forward-head posture increases the compressive force between the facet articular cartilage of the inferior articular process and the adjacent facet of the superior articular process. Maintenance of this posture for prolonged periods does not allow for the cyclic compression and decompression needed to maintain cartilage health.

Because the repair capabilities of articular cartilage are minimal, cyclic compression and decompression become even more critical. This is especially relevant when considering cervical spondylosis. In simple terms, spondylosis refers to

Table 1–2. Comparative Coefficients of Friction		
	Lubricant	Coefficient of Friction
Nylon on steel	None	0.300
Graphite on graphite	None	0.100
Steel on steel	Oil	0.050
Plastic on metal (total hip)	SF	0.060
Teflon on Teflon	None	0.050
Metal on cartilage (Austin Moore)	SF	0.032
Skate on ice	H_2O	0.030
Steel on ice	None	0.030
Cartilage on cartilage	SF	0.005

SF, Synovial fluid.

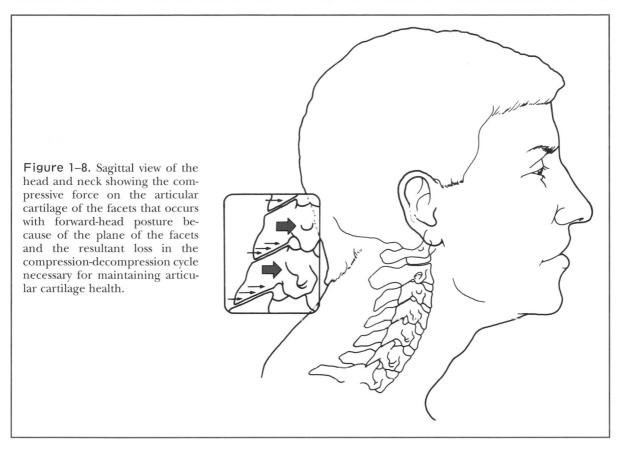

Figure 1–8. Sagittal view of the head and neck showing the compressive force on the articular cartilage of the facets that occurs with forward-head posture because of the plane of the facets and the resultant loss in the compression-decompression cycle necessary for maintaining articular cartilage health.

the degenerative process of the spine (the mechanism of which is described below), and the syndrome includes not only the degenerative changes that occur at the intervertebral disc, but those that occur at the articular cartilage of the apophyseal joint as well. In the presence of such a degenerative process, pain frequently is unresolved over the long term because the joint pathology is a chronic process. Therefore, the only rational therapy for abnormalities within the joint includes exercise programs that offer stabilization of the range of motion by muscle activity and improved nutrition of the joint by mechanical activity.[31]

The degeneration of articular cartilage places increasing stress on the subchondral bone. As the cartilage fibrillates and gradually thins, it loses elasticity. The subchondral bone then begins to take up the increased load. Bony sclerosis and osteophytes are the eventual sequelae of this process (Fig. 1–9).

Noncontractile Supporting Tissues: Ligaments, Fascia, and Intervertebral Disc

Noncontractile supporting tissues provide stability between the bones and at the same time allow mobility in specific directions. These tissues offer support primarily because of their viscoelastic qualities. Viscoelasticity often is represented by a spring-and-dashpot mechanism, which suggests that within a specified range of stress, the tissue has elasticity that allows it to return to its original shape but at the same time is resistant to deformation (Fig. 1–10).

The capacity of these support tissues to elongate and remain permanently elongated is limited and probably varies with different areas of the body and among individuals. The stress-strain curve (see Fig. 1–5) shows the elongation capacity for connective tissues and the point at which

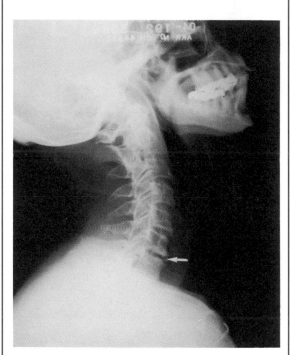

Figure 1–9. Radiographs of the cervical spine showing a loss of apophyseal joint space and the resultant bone spurs.

connective tissues begin microtearing and frank rupture occurs.

Whereas loading of the tissues can be graphically depicted with the stress-strain curve, the unloading of tissues is not simply a reversal of the loading pattern. In fact, restoration to the original length of the tissue after stretch occurs at a lesser rate and often to a lesser extent than elongation. The loss of energy between the lengthening force and the recovery activity is termed hys-

teresis (Fig. 1–11). As more chemical bonds are broken with an elongation force, the greater the hysteresis and the resulting new set point become for the tissues. The new set point is especially important when it affects the supporting ligaments of the spine because stability between adjacent vertebra elements is lost, which allows for aberrational translational movements between segments.

Connective tissue structures can offer stability only when the collagen framework is subject to tension. Periodic, nondestructive loading patterns strengthen and thicken these support tissues.[39]

The optimal health of various elements of the specialized connective tissue system is partially related to the tissues' ability to effectively load and unload within their physiological capacity. High-impact loads and prolonged loading stress these tissues in ranges beyond their physiological capacity for tolerance and result in injury and altered function.

NEUROMUSCULAR SYSTEM

The muscles direct forces through the specialized connective tissues by way of their attachments to the various bony levers. The actions of muscles related to the cervical spine ultimately depend on the afferent information supplied from the joint and muscle receptors and the special receptors associated with the head. An especially sophisticated afferent-efferent network of neuromuscular reflexes is integrated with the cervical spine because of profuse reflex connections with the auditory, visual, and vestibular apparati.

Muscle activity helps to counterbalance the forces of gravity and movement and allows for movement patterns that minimize abnormal

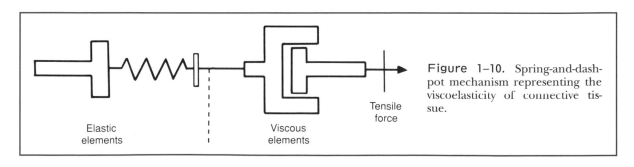

Elastic elements

Viscous elements

Tensile force

Figure 1–10. Spring-and-dashpot mechanism representing the viscoelasticity of connective tissue.

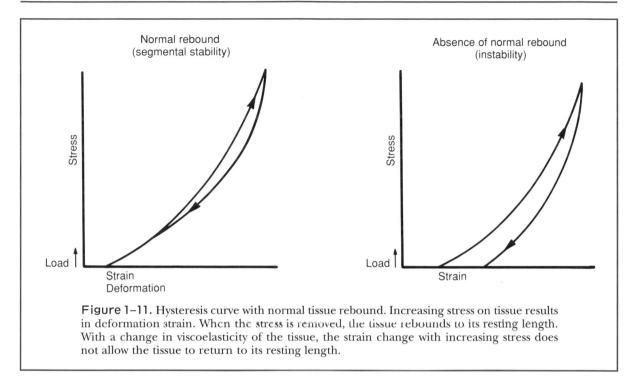

Figure 1–11. Hysteresis curve with normal tissue rebound. Increasing stress on tissue results in deformation strain. When the stress is removed, the tissue rebounds to its resting length. With a change in viscoelasticity of the tissue, the strain change with increasing stress does not allow the tissue to return to its resting length.

stresses to elements of the specialized connective tissues. Such precise control and discrete function of the neuromuscular system allow a shock absorption function to be attributed to muscles. When the central nervous system is presented with nociceptive stimuli, there is increased control of movement patterns, which restricts available motion and force transference through injured tissues. The neuromuscular system thus plays an important role in directing potentially destructive forces away from an injured area.

Several significant afferent sources in addition to the joint and muscle receptor system need to be mentioned to fully comprehend the multiplicity of factors that can affect the resting state of muscle tension. This is especially relevant in a discussion of cervical spine disorders because many emotional and environmental stimuli contribute to the status of muscle resting tension in patients with cervical spine pain (Fig. 1–12). Factors include injury and inflammation as well as such stresses as temperature, diet, pattern of sleep, and emotional state. The treatment of upper-quarter problems often is geared toward minimizing the afferent input into the central ner-

vous system and assisting patients to recognize the relation between those accumulated stimuli and their current condition. A primary consideration in mechanical neck pain is the psychological factors that contribute to the painful syndrome.

PSYCHOSOCIAL ASPECTS OF CERVICAL SPINE DISORDERS

In broad terms, any afferent stimulus that impacts on the central nervous system can be termed a stress. Stress has been defined as any stimulus that causes the body to react.[36] Most stimuli cause at least some level of response, whether it be from one organ or a complete system. As an example, a certain stimulus may elicit low-grade muscle contraction or diffuse sympathetic nervous system activation.

Pain in the neck is one of the more debilitating musculoskeletal problems. Painless, unrestricted mobility of the neck is a prerequisite for many occupational, recreational, and social functions. Because of the elaborate sensory system of the

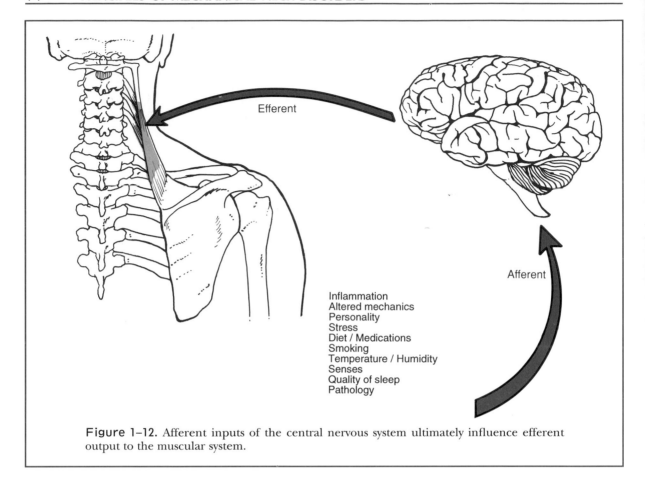

Efferent

Afferent

Inflammation
Altered mechanics
Personality
Stress
Diet / Medications
Smoking
Temperature / Humidity
Senses
Quality of sleep
Pathology

Figure 1–12. Afferent inputs of the central nervous system ultimately influence efferent output to the muscular system.

head, the neck is active in nearly every activity, from simple activities such as nodding and shaking hands to more complex ones such as tracking an object flying through the air. A disruption of neck function can have a significant impact on the activities of daily living or on occupational demands.

Complaints of neck pain can be influenced by psychological, emotional, social, and cultural factors unique to the patient. The head, neck, and face are musculoskeletal regions in which stressors often manifest themselves. More than a clinician realizes, the evaluation of a patient is essentially the weighing and assessment of the importance of anatomical, pathological, mechanical, and psychological factors that contribute to the painful syndrome.[33] Not only must dysfunction of the neck, shoulder girdle, head, and face be evalu-

ated, but the psychological factors that influence the problem must be addressed. The clinician must assess both the pathomechanical and the emotional contributions to the complaint. Psychological factors are of special significance because of their relevance to chronic pain syndrome.

An understanding of psychosocial factors is central to comprehensive management of the painful neck syndrome because being able to separate acute pain from chronic pain is important for cost-effective and responsible care. Waddell's observations regarding the difference between acute and chronic pain in the low back are directly applicable to neck pain:

Acute and chronic pain are not only different in time scale but are fundamentally different in kind. Acute pain bears a relatively straightforward relationship to peripheral stimulus, nociception, and tissue damage. There may be some understandable anxiety about the meaning and consequences of the pain, but acute pain, acute disability, and acute illness behavior are generally proportionate to the physical findings. Pharmacologic, physical, and even surgical treatments directed to the underlying physical disorder are generally highly effective in relieving acute pain. In contrast, chronic pain, chronic disability, and chronic illness behavior become increasingly dissociated from their original physical basis, and there may indeed be little objective evidence of any remaining nociceptive stimulus. Instead, chronic pain and disability become increasingly associated with emotional distress, depression, failed treatment, and adoption of a sick role. Chronic pain progressively becomes a self-sustaining condition that is resistant to traditional medical management. Physical treatment directed to a supposed but unidentified and possibly nonexistent nociceptive source is not only understandably unsuccessful but failed treatment may both reinforce and aggravate pain, distress, disability, and illness behavior.[42]

Thus, the distinction between acute and chronic pain is not quantitative but rather qualitative, and the means to assess chronic pain behavior is of fundamental importance for the clinician.[6] An overview of the contributions of illness behavior and emotional disorders to chronic neck pain follows. For a more comprehensive review, the reader is referred to other sources.[5, 33, 35]

Illness Behavior

Illness behavior reflects the patient's conscious or unconscious desire to communicate pain or suffering, albeit from physical or psychological dysfunction or a combination of these. Inappropriate illness behaviors are coping responses that are out of proportion to the physical stimulus of injury.

Coping responses that allow the clinician to recognize signs of illness behavior include excessive use of medications, especially narcotics and tranquilizers; excessive grimacing, groaning, holding, or rubbing of the injured body part; anatomical descriptions of pain that defy known referred pain patterns; and excessive use of multiple health care providers. Inappropriate illness behavior also encompasses irresponsible use of the reward contingencies that are operating in the patient's life, such as work avoidance, social interaction avoidance, and financial gain.

Questions should be asked during the history in an attempt to ascertain such information. Listening closely and carefully observing the patient during the interview are the first steps in assessing the contribution of psychological factors to the painful syndrome. The patient uses verbal and nonverbal behaviors to appeal for attention and support from family, co-workers, and the clinician.

Emotional Disorders

Assessing the contribution of a patient's emotional state to his particular disorder is a challenging task because in fact many emotions are an appropriate response to pain. The clinician should be particularly cognizant of such emotional states as excessive anxiety, anger, hostility, and depression.

The history portion of the examination affords an opportunity to assess the patient's anxiety and depression levels. Depression is common in patients with chronic pain either because of the suffering that has occurred as a result of the syndrome or because of preexisting traits that magnify the discomfort or its consequences. A useful rule of thumb for the clinician is that anxious patients make the interviewer anxious and depressed patients make the interviewer sad.[25]

Awareness of these emotional states is especially important because of their influence on the neuromuscular system. Many cervical spine disorders have a component of muscle guarding, spasm, and pain, and the emotional state must be carefully weighed because it promulgates the painful or dysfunctional syndrome (Fig. 1–13). Emotional states also evoke sympathetic nervous system activity, and such discharge exacerbates and maintains the painful state.[9] Nociceptors are further excited by an increase in sympathetic nervous system activity and the presence of released norepinephrine.[19] Patients who consider their neck pain unbearable often elicit a protective autonomic response that is disproportionate to the original stimulus. Although chronic pain of the neck is certainly disconcerting, it is, by definition, bearable because the patient has had it for many months.[33]

Stressors in a person's life may come from several sources: environmental, social, psychological, physical. Successful management of a patient

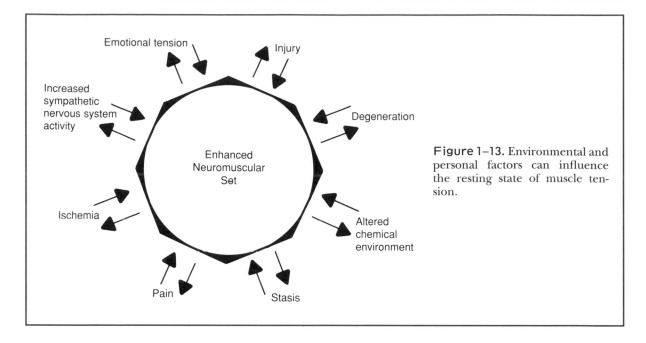

Figure 1–13. Environmental and personal factors can influence the resting state of muscle tension.

with chronic neck pain in whom stress contributes to the syndrome includes identifying the stressor and then altering the stressor itself, the patient's perception of the stress, or the patient's response to the stress. Dissecting the psychological contribution from the physical symptom is a daunting task but a necessary one so that inappropriate treatment strategies are avoided. To focus on pain modulation or pain relief with patients who show evidence of psychological dysfunction legitimates their complaint and reinforces symptom magnification. Restoration or improvement of function becomes a more realistic goal.

RELATING THE PRINCIPLES OF MECHANICAL NECK PAIN TO CERVICAL SPINE DISORDERS

In most conditions, it is difficult to identify the exact tissue that may be at fault with cervical disorders, and the reality is that most syndromes probably involve several tissues or structures. As a result, a plethora of syndromes and diagnoses for neck problems has emerged, often largely influenced by examiner bias.

The most common causes of neck pain are the locking or painful neck with accompanying spasmodic torticollis, muscle and connective tissue strain occurring as a result of postural overload or repetitive motion, injuries resulting from uncontrolled acceleration of the head and neck, and cervical spondylosis.

As a means of applying several concepts discussed earlier in this chapter, acceleration injury and cervical spondylosis are discussed further. These clinical entities provide a framework of reference for many mechanical disorders of the neck, and specific syndromes commonly bear elements of one or both. This discussion also provides a useful clinical reference for subsequent discussions regarding the neurosciences, articulations, and muscles related to the cervical spine.

Acceleration Injury of the Cervical Spine

The term *acceleration injury* is used rather than *whiplash* because it is more inclusive and descriptive of the injury mechanisms that potentially result in rapid acceleration and deceleration of the cervical spine. Motor vehicle accidents are a major cause of acceleration injury. This type of injury is especially difficult to manage because in addition to affecting the musculoskeletal tissues, it can lead to the involvement of several other anatomical regions, such as the central nervous system, esophagus, trachea, and temporomandibular joint.

Radanov and colleagues have suggested a clinically useful separation of acceleration injuries into cervicoencephalic and cervicobrachial groupings, which recognizes the functional anatomy of the upper and lower cervical spine.[34] The cervicoencephalic syndrome classification recognizes the intimate relation between the occiput–cervical spine complex and the brain, brain stem, and spinal cord. Symptoms from acceleration injuries resulting in cervicoencephalic syndromes might include headache, fatigue, vertigo, poor concentration, irritability to noise and light, and cognitive dysfunction as well as neck pain. These symptoms imply that in addition to the musculoskeletal tissues being damaged with the acceleration injury, the central nervous system structures are injured, which leads to neuro-psychophysiological disturbances (Table 1–3).

Among the most taxing and challenging features of acceleration injury of the neck is *Barré syndrome.* Symptoms of this syndrome include suboccipital headache, vertigo, tinnitus, intermittent aphonia and hoarseness, fatigue, temperature changes, and dysesthesias of the hands and forearms provoked by emotion, temperature, humidity, or noise. Craniofacial complaints also occur with associated pain, numbness, nausea, vomiting, and, occasionally, diarrhea. These symptoms are considered to arise from hypertonia of the sympathetic nervous system. This condition may result from stretch injury and hemorrhage within the sympathetic chain ganglia or by irritation of the ventral roots from C5-T1, all of which contain sympathetic fibers.[24]

Cervicobrachial disorders feature neck pain with upper-extremity pain, whether the syndrome is characterized by neck pain greater than extremity pain or extremity pain greater than neck pain. In either case, the implication is that in addition to the musculoskeletal tissues of the cervical spine being injured, referred pain from the injured cervical tissues or radicular pain from lesions of the nerve root complex accompanies the neck disorder.

This is an anatomically useful classification because it implies that the cervicoencephalic disorder is more closely related to upper cervical spine disturbances, whereas the cervico-brachial disorder is related to lower cervical spine disturbances. A precise, detailed history that assesses pain location, symptomatology, and magnitude of forces causing the injury is essential. Passive motion testing and palpation, as reviewed in Chapter 5, can then be used to substantiate the information typically gained in the history. In any event, the pathomechanics of the specialized connective tissues and muscles and the response of the neuromuscular system to the injury are the focus of the clinician.

There is a marked difference in the outcome of acceleration injuries, depending on whether the imparted force results in an excessive and rapid hyperextension motion or a hyperflexion motion of the head and neck. Hyperextension forces that occur in an acceleration injury cause an excessive range of motion for the cervical spine because the abrupt stop to the motion occurs only when the occiput contacts the posterior thorax (Fig. 1–14). A hyperflexion injury typically does not move the neck through a comparable range of motion because the chin strikes the chest or, if there is a lateral flexion component, the ear contacts the shoulder. Macnab has noted that acceleration injuries that result in chronic neck pain are nearly always caused by hyperextension forces.[30]

In an acceleration injury, excessive shear and tensile forces are exerted on the cervical spine. With an understanding of the science of soft tissue healing and results of injury to the physiological loading capacity of tissues as noted above, the clinician can teach initial positions of rest (decreased tension and shear) during the early stages of healing, followed by the introduction of controlled passive and active motions (gradual reintroduction of stress to tissues), and then progress to teaching patterns of movement to

Table 1–3. Symptoms of Cervicoencephalic Syndrome
Cerebral concussion
Barré syndrome (sympathetic dysfunction)
Cranial nerve dysfunction
Headache
Cognitive impairment

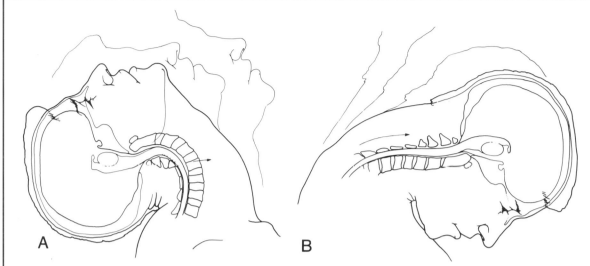

Figure 1–14. Excessive range of motion that occurs with hyperextension injuries compared with the range of motion with flexion injuries. The occiput hits the posterior thorax with hyperextension *(A)*, whereas the chin hits the chest with hyperflexion *(B)*. Because the hyperextension excursion is so much greater, the anterior structures of the neck are especially vulnerable with acceleration injury.

minimize excessive stresses to the injured region while establishing realistic short- and long-term goals.

Cervical Spondylosis

Cervical spondylosis presents the most comprehensive example of the degenerative process and age-related changes of the cervical spine leading to mechanical neck pain. Cervical spondylosis typically is defined as the age-related, degenerative changes that begin at the intervertebral disk and subsequently involve other tissues, such as the articular cartilage of the apophyseal joints, and the bones of the cervical spine, including the unciform processes. The involvement of multiple tissues in the syndrome presents a clear example of how the aging process alters the physiological loading capacity of the cervical spine. In its broadest sense, cervical spondylosis is degeneration of the cervical spine.

As with acceleration injury, it is useful to divide the clinical presentation of cervical spondylosis into meaningful groupings (Table 1–4). An understanding of the degenerative process and the resulting sequelae of symptoms and signs suggests that four clinical subgroups of spondylosis should be recognized: neck pain, neck pain with referral, radicular pain, and myelopathy.

Cervical spondylitic myelopathy, which is compromise of the spinal cord within the spinal canal as a result of degenerative changes of the cervical spine, is the most serious consequence of cervical intervertebral disc degeneration and the most common cervical spinal cord disorder after middle age.[27, 43]

Pathogenesis

The pathological process of cervical spondylosis begins with a decrease in hydration and in the water-binding capacity of the nucleus pulposus. This change in hydration capacity typically

Table 1–4. Symptoms of Cervical Spondylosis
Neck pain
Neck pain with proximal referral
Radicular pain
Myelopathy

begins during the third decade. Because the decrease in hydration lessens the intradiscal pressure—the pressure exerted by the hydrophilic nucleus pulposus against the inner walls of the annulus fibrosus—tension cannot be maintained within the annular rings and they buckle as they become excessively loaded in compression (see Chapter 4). As a result, the annulus fibrosus fibrillates and weakens. The margins of the optimal loading zone for the intervertebral disc are now altered.

As the disc loses its structural integrity, the adjacent vertebral bodies become approximated. As a result, a reactive process occurs in the bones of the cervical spine, with osteophytes developing along the peripheral attachments of the intervertebral disc to the vertebral body. The development of osteophytes also occurs at the joints of Luschka and the apophyseal joints. Posterior osteophytes along the margins of the vertebral body decrease the sagittal diameter of the spinal canal and present potential regions of mechanical compromise to the spinal cord or nerve root complex. Osteophytes that develop on the anterior aspect of the vertebral body may compress the esophagus. Disc-space narrowing, the formation of osteophytes, and sclerosing of the vertebral bodies are typical changes seen in the pathogenesis of cervical spondylosis.

The other key element of the specialized connective tissues, the articular cartilage of the apophyseal joints, also undergoes significant degenerative change. Loss of the joint space as a result of fibrillation and erosion of the articular cartilage occurs. Without articular cartilage to attenuate the forces of compression and shear, the subchondral bone of the articular facet undergoes a reactive phase. Bony sclerosis and osteophytes are typical changes seen at the apophyseal joints in cervical spondylosis. These osteophytes have the potential to compromise the nerve root complex as it exits from the intervertebral foramen.

Although the pathogenesis of the spondylosis process can be described and such changes clearly alter the mobility of the cervical spine and reduce its force-attenuating capability, there is not a clear correlation between structural changes and symptoms. Several studies have noted that there is little difference between structural changes of symptomatic and asymptomatic patients.[11, 16, 41] It is, therefore, essential that the degenerative changes are correlated with the signs and symptoms presented clinically.

An understanding of the aging and degenerative processes of the cervical spine is important to set realistic short- and long-term goals in the management of mechanical neck pain. Although we have little information allowing for a clear differentiation between age-related changes and the degenerative process of the cervical spine, we do understand that altered function is the end result of both processes.

SUMMARY

This textbook details the functional anatomy of the cervical spine, and it develops an assessment and treatment approach based on the science of tissue repair and the response of tissues to controlled therapeutic stresses. Neck pain problems are a significant source of disability to patients, but they have not been studied as extensively as low back pain problems. A review of the prevalence and incidence of neck disorders provides some understanding of the impact of the problem. In many mechanical neck disorders, the tissues at fault cannot be identified, and a painful syndrome probably results from the involvement of several different tissues. For this reason, analyses of the mechanics of injury and of the stresses that reproduce the familiar syndrome provide the clinician with a basis for setting goals and developing a treatment program. To fully understand the scope of symptoms and signs that accompany neck disorders, it is important to have a fundamental knowledge of the impact of psychological stress, emotional disorders, and illness behaviors. Finally, it is essential for the clinician dealing with mechanical neck pain to understand the components of the specialized connective tissue system and the response of the neuromuscular system to injury.

REFERENCES

1. Andersson GBJ: Epidemiology of spinal disorders. *In* Frymoyer J (ed): The Adult Spine. New York, Raven Press, 1991, p 137.

2. Aryanpur J, Ducker TB: Differential diagnosis and management of cervical spine pain. *In* Tollison CD (ed): Handbook of Chronic Pain Management. Baltimore, Williams & Wilkins, 1989, pp 320–334.
3. Bennett GJ: The role of the sympathetic nervous system in painful peripheral neuropathy. Pain 45:221–223, 1991.
4. Cailliet R: Pain: Mechanisms and Management. Philadelphia, FA Davis, 1993, pp 99–123.
5. Chapman CR, Bonica JJ: Chronic Pain. Kalamazoo, MI, Upjohn, 1985.
6. DeRosa C, Porterfield JA: A physical therapy model for the treatment of low back pain. Phys Ther 72:261–272, 1992.
7. Deyo RA, Tsui-Wu YJ: Descriptive terminology of low back pain and its related medical care in the United States. Spine 12:264–268, 1987.
8. Dvorak J, Valach L, Schmidt S: Cervical spine injuries in Switzerland. J Manual Med 4:7–16, 1989.
9. Faulkner JA, Niemeyer JH, Maxwell LC, et al: Contractile properties of transplanted extensor digitorum longus muscles in cats. Am J Physiol 238:C120–C126, 1980.
10. Feldenkrais M: Body and Mature Behavior. New York, International University Press, 1973.
11. Friedenberg ZB, Miller WY: Degenerative disc disease of the cervical spine. J Bone Joint Surg [Am] 45A:1171–1179, 1963.
12. Garret WE Jr, Seaber AV, Boswick J, et al: Recovery of skeletal muscle after laceration and repair. J Hand Surg 9A:683–692, 1984.
13. Gay JR, Abbott KH: Common whiplash injuries of the neck. JAMA 152:1698–1704, 1953.
14. Gotten N: Survey of one hundred cases of whiplash injury after settlement of litigation. JAMA 162:865–867, 1956.
15. Gower WE, Pedrim V: Age related variation in protein polysaccharides from human nucleus pulposus, annulus fibrosus, and costal cartilage. J Bone Joint Surg [Am] 51A:1154–1162, 1969.
16. Hiltsberger WE, Witten R: Abnormal myelograms in asymptomatic patients. J Neurosurg 28:204, 1968.
17. Hirsch C, Paulson S, Sylven B, Snellman O: Biophysical and physiological investigation on cartilage and other mesenchymal tissues; characteristics of human nuclei pulposi during aging. Acta Orthop Scand 22:175–183, 1953.
18. Hocking B: Epidemiological aspects of repetitive strain injury in Telecom, Australia. Med J Aust 147:218–222, 1987.
19. Hu S, Zhu J: Sympathetic facilitation of sustained discharges of polymodal nociceptors. Pain 38:85–90, 1989.
20. Hult L: Cervical, dorsal, and lumbar spine syndromes. Acta Orthop Scand Suppl 17:1–102, 1954.
21. Keisler S, Finholt T: The mystery of RSI. Am Psychol 43:1004–1015, 1988.
22. Kelsey JL, Githens PB, Walter SD, et al: An epidemiologic study of acute prolapsed intervertebral disc. J Bone Joint Surg [Am] 66:907–914, 1984.
23. Kondo K, Molgaard CA, Kurland LT, Onofrio BM: Protruded intervertebral disc. Minn Med 64:751–753, 1981.
24. LaRocca H: Cervical sprain syndrome. *In* Frymoyer J (ed): The Adult Spine. New York, Raven Press, 1991, p 1055.
25. Liang MH, Katz JN: Clinical evaluation of patients with a suspected spine problem. *In* Frymoyer J (ed): The Adult Spine. New York, Raven Press, 1991, p 223.
26. Lieberman JS: Cervical soft tissue injuries and cervical disc disease. *In* Lieberman JS (ed): Principles of Physical Medicine and Rehabilitation in the Musculoskeletal Diseases. New York, Grune & Stratton, 1986, pp 263–286.
27. Lundsford LD, Bissonette DJ, Zorub DS: Anterior surgery for cervical disc disease. II. Treatment of cervical spondylotic myelopathy in 32 cases. J Neurosurg 53:12–19, 1980.
28. McDermott FT: Repetition strain injury: A review of current understanding. Med J Aust 144:196–200, 1986.
29. Macnab I: Acceleration injuries of the cervical spine. *In* Symposium on the Spine. St. Louis, CV Mosby, 1969, pp 10–17.
30. Macnab I: Acceleration injuries of the cervical spine. J Bone Joint Surg [Am] 46:1797–1799, 1964.
31. Mooney V: The facet syndrome. *In* Weinstein JN, Wiesel SW (eds): The Lumbar Spine. Philadelphia, WB Saunders, 1990, pp 422–440.
32. Norris SH, Watt I: The prognosis of neck injuries resulting from rear end collisions. J Bone Joint Surg [Br] 65:608–611, 1983.
33. Ciccone DS, Grzesiak CD: Psychological dysfunction in chronic neck pain. *In* Tollison CD, Sofferthwaite JR (eds): Painful Cervical Trauma. Baltimore, Williams & Wilkins, 1992, pp 79–92.
34. Radanov BP, Dvorak J, Valach L: Cognitive deficits in patients after soft tissue injury of the cervical spine. Spine 17:127–131, 1992.
35. Sarno JE: Etiology of neck and back and neck pain an autonomic myoneuralgia. J Nerv Ment Dis 169:55–59, 1981.
36. Selye H: The Stress of Life. New York, McGraw-Hill, 1956.
37. Severy DM, Mathewson JH, Bechtol CO: Controlled automobile rear-end collisions: An investigation of related engineering and medical phenomena. Can Services Med J 11:717–759, 1955.
38. Shephard RJ: Physical Activity and Aging. Chicago, Year Book Medical, 1978, pp 44–50.
39. Stone MH: Implications for connective tissue and bone alterations resulting from resistance exercise training. Med Sci Sports Exerc 20:5(Suppl):S162–S168, 1988.
40. Takala J, Sievers K, Klaukka T: Rheumatic symptoms in the middle aged population in southwestern Finland. Scand J Rheumatol Suppl 47:15–29, 1982.
41. Tapiovarra J, Heinivaara O: Correlation of cervico-brachialgias and roentgenographic findings. Ann Chir Gynaecol Suppl 43:436, 1954.
42. Waddell G: A new clinical model for the treatment of low back pain. Spine 12:632–644, 1987.
43. Wilberger JE, Chedid MK: Acute cervical spondylotic myelopathy. Neurosurgery 22:145–146, 1988.
44. Woo SL-Y, Inoue M, McGurk-Burleson E, et al: Treatment of the medial collateral ligament. II. Structure and function of canine knees in response to differing treatment regimens. Am J Sports Med 15:22–29, 1987.

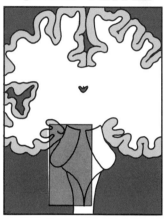

CHAPTER 2

NEUROPHYSIOLOGICAL IMPLICATIONS OF MECHANICAL NECK PAIN

The neurosciences related to the head and cervical spine present a degree of complexity unique in the axial skeleton. Despite this intricacy, the application of neuroanatomy and neurophysiology to clinical disorders that affect the neck is necessary in classifying the nature of the syndrome. In addition to an understanding of nerve root dysfunction, the clinician often is required to assess or, at the minimum, rule out spinal cord and brain stem involvement.

Several unique features of the neurosciences related to the cervical spine are immediately apparent. They include the following:

1. The transitional region between the lower portion of the brain stem and the beginning of the spinal cord within the cervical spinal canal

2. A nerve root complex featuring an extended route of exit to the periphery through the lateral recess of the spinal canal and intervertebral foramen and coursing in proximity to the vertebral artery

3. The sympathetic chain housed in the walls of the carotid sheath and traveling the length of the anterolateral cervical spine

4. Descending brain stem motor tracts such as the tectospinal and medial vestibulospinal that do not reach any other areas of the spinal cord ex-

cept the cervical and are intimately associated with reflex motor activity of the head and neck

5. Reflex connections between the special senses of sight and hearing and the ventral horn cells that innervate the cervical spine musculature

6. Intricate reflex loops linking the vestibular apparatus, extraocular muscles, and muscles of the head and neck

These and other features suggest neuroanatomical and neurophysiological characteristics that have a profound influence on the head and neck function. Because many painful syndromes of the upper quarter require an assessment of neurological function, this chapter provides an overview of the neuroanatomy relevant to cervical spine function and the neuromechanical and neurochemical basis of cervical spine disorders.

GROSS MORPHOLOGY OF THE SPINAL CANAL AND ITS CONTENTS

The spinal cord, meningeal coverings (dura, arachnoid, pia mater), and nerve root complex are all housed within the spinal canal. When the posterior muscles have been dissected from their

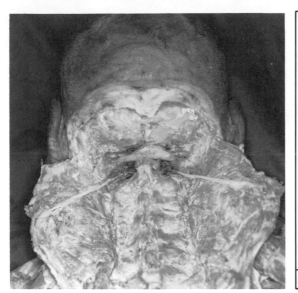 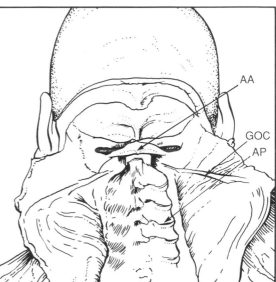

Figure 2–1. Posterior aspect of the cervical spine. The suboccipital muscles and remaining deep cervical muscles have been removed. The spinal cord is seen just inferior to the arch of the atlas. The joint capsules of the cervical apophyseal joints on the right have been removed to allow for identification of the articular pillars. AA, arch of the atlas; AP, articular pillar; GOC, greater occipital nerve.

vertebral attachments, the detail of the bony and ligamentous housing for these central nervous system structures can be appreciated (Fig. 2–1).

The posterior walls of the spinal canal are formed by the midline spinous process and the two adjacent lamina of the vertebral arch. From the lamina, the ligamentum flavum courses to the adjacent vertebrae, effectively contributing to the formation of the posterior wall of the spinal canal. The posterior boundary of the spinal canal is thus formed by bony and ligamentous tissue.

The lateral recess of the spinal canal is an important area because it represents the location of a significant portion of the nerve root complex. The primary bony elements that contribute to the formation of the lateral recess are the pedicles, which feature bony channels on their superior surfaces in which the exiting nerve roots travel. The medial aspect of the articular pillars is also intimately related to the lateral recess, with the inferior facet more closely approximating the spinal canal than the superior facet.

Anterolaterally, the wall of the spinal canal is formed by raised lateral ridges of the vertebral body known as the unciform processes. As two adjacent vertebrae approximate and the unciform processes articulate with the inferior aspect of the adjacent vertebrae, the unciform joints (also referred to as the joints of Luschka) are formed. These joints help to serve as anterolateral borders of the spinal canal. Lastly, the posterior aspect of the vertebral body, intervertebral disk, and wide posterior longitudinal ligament compose the anterior wall of the spinal canal.

The contents of the spinal canal can be exposed by removing the posterior wall of the spinal canal (i.e., the spinous process and both lamina with the attached ligamentum flavum). In Figure 2–2, the spinal canal as well as the apophyseal joints on the left side have been removed to follow the nerve root complex. The apophyseal joints have been left intact on the left side to recognize the relation of the nerve root complex to the joints. The dural covering of the spinal cord and nerve root remains intact when this approach is used.

The dura, arachnoid, and pia mater cover the spinal cord and nerve root complex, but only the dura can be immediately seen when the posterior wall of the spinal canal is removed. The dura mater lines the spinal canal and is separated from the periosteum by fat and veins in the epidural space. The dura forms a tent-like funnel through which the nerve roots penetrate on their path through the intervertebral foramen. The tent-like arrangement of the dura with its apex directed laterally toward the intervertebral foramen helps the nerve root avoid being pulled through the intervertebral foramen because the dura plugs the foramen when a tensile force is placed on the nerve root complex by way of the peripheral nerves.[31] The potential for avulsion of the cervical nerve roots is lessened by such an anatomical arrangement. The dorsal root ganglion is also covered with this dural investment.

Lining the internal aspect of the dura mater is the delicate arachnoid membrane. Since the arachnoid is attached to the inner dura, wide spaces are created where the dura and arachnoid are separated from the pia mater and medullary contents (spinal cord and nerve root tissue). Because the pia mater remains closely invested to the medullary contents of the spinal canal, the subarachnoid space is created in which the cerebrospinal fluid is housed. In specific regions of the spinal canal, the pia mater is thickened to form dentate ligaments that course through the subarachnoid space to attach to the arachnoid and dura to anchor and help suspend the spinal cord in the spinal canal.

BIOMECHANICS OF THE SPINAL CORD

The relationship between the upper cervical spinal canal and the spinal cord is unique. There is more free space for the spinal cord in the upper two cervical segments than anywhere else in the spine (Fig. 2–3).[34] Proceeding caudally in the spinal canal, there is less free space between the spinal cord and the spinal canal.

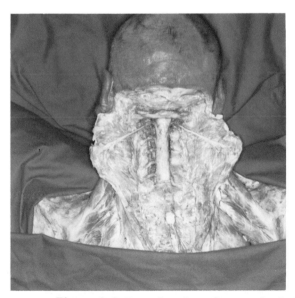
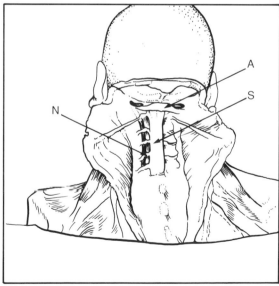

Figure 2–2. Posterior view of exposed spinal canal with dura intact over the spinal cord and nerve roots. The apophyseal joints have been kept intact on the right side but have been removed on the left side, which allows for exposure of the nerve root complex. A, atlas; N, nerve root complex with dural sheath and dorsal root ganglion; S, spinal cord and dural covering.

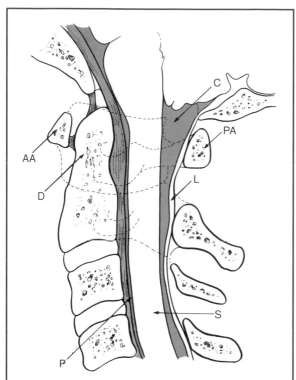

Figure 2–3. Sagittal view of cervical spine showing a greater degree of free space for the spinal cord in the upper two cervical segments than in the lower cervical segments. Just posterior to the upper cervical cord and lower brain stem is the large cisterna magna. AA, anterior arch of atlas (cut); C, cisterna magna; D, dens; L, ligamentum flavum; P, posterior longitudinal ligament; PA, posterior arch of atlas; S, spinal cord.

The spinal canal can be considered dynamic in the sense that its dimensions are altered with spinal motion. The length and cross-sectional area of the spinal canal change during flexion, extension, and lateral bending of the cervical spine. These changes in canal dimensions require a degree of accommodation by the spinal cord and meningeal coverings.

Extension of the cervical spine decreases the sagittal diameter of the vertebral canal. Extension also allows the ligamentum flavum to retract and thicken by redistribution of its volume. This is clinically relevant because a hypertrophic ligamentum flavum that might occur as a sequelae to the degenerative process and buckling of the ligamentum flavum during cervical extension can decrease the sagittal diameter of the spinal canal. This decrease in sagittal diameter, especially at the middle and lower cervical regions, can potentially compromise the spinal cord.

When the cervical spine is extended, the spinal cord begins to resemble an accordion being squeezed toward closing, with folds detectable on the posterior surface of the spinal cord and dura mater at full extension (Fig. 2–4). When the cervical spine is flexed, the spinal cord as well as the nerve roots and their meningeal coverings are subjected to tensile stresses. The spinal canal is relatively longer in flexion than in extension because the center of rotation for sagittal plane motion of the cervical spine lies anterior to the spinal canal (Fig. 2–5). This requires an elongation of all structures posterior to this center of rotation. Because of its placement relative to this center of rotation, the spinal cord lengthens and thins with flexion and shortens and thickens with extension.[20]

Tensile forces in the spinal cord generated as a result of elongation are attenuated primarily by the meningeal coverings and secondarily by the cord itself. Tensile forces imparted to the cord are further balanced by tangential tensile forces from the nerve root complex and the anchoring mechanism of the filum terminale. The tangential forces exerted by the nerve root complex are transmitted to the cord predominantly through the nerve root dural sheaths and dentate ligaments rather than by the roots and rootlets themselves.[20]

Maximum stretching of the neural elements occurs between C2 and T1.[28] With a large posterior central disk protrusion, the spinal cord and meningeal coverings are subjected not only to this tensile stress, but to a compressive force of the intervertebral disk on the anterior aspect of the spinal cord as well.

These mechanics of the spinal cord suggest that its structure is inherently flexible. This flexibility is not readily appreciated because of its extensive anchoring within the spinal canal. Dural attachments to each of the subpedicular recesses, nerve root sheaths, and dentate ligaments; the continuation of the spinal cord with the medulla of the brain stem; and suspension by way of the filum terminale attachment all help to provide

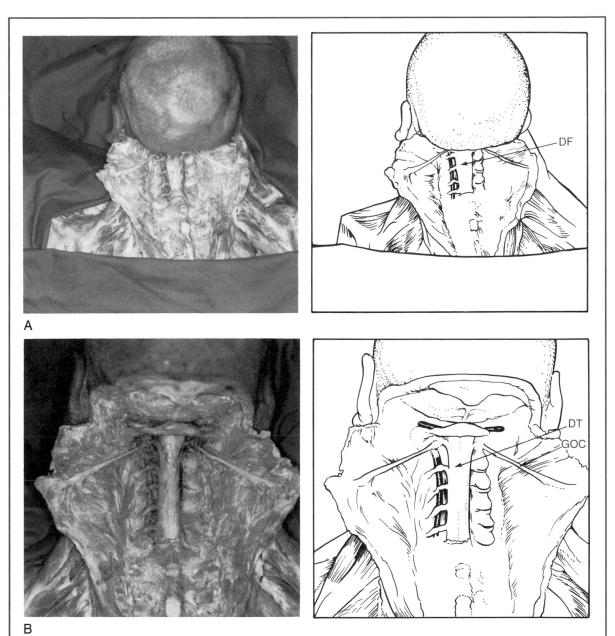

Figure 2–4. *A,* The occiput and cervical spine are extended, which causes a folding of the dura and the spinal cord. *B,* A flexion force places a tension force on the dura and the spinal cord. DF, dura folded with extension; DT, tension on dura with flexion; GOC, greater occipital nerve.

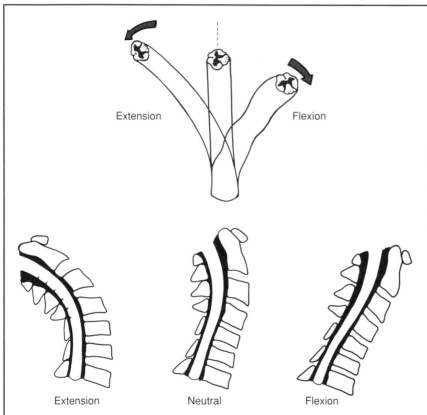

Figure 2–5. Folding and unfolding characteristics of the spinal cord during extension and flexion. Because the axis of motion for flexion and extension lies anterior to the neuroaxis, elongation is required when flexion occurs. As flexion proceeds, the spinal cord begins to unfold and then undergoes elastic deformation. During extension, the spinal cord is relatively shortened.

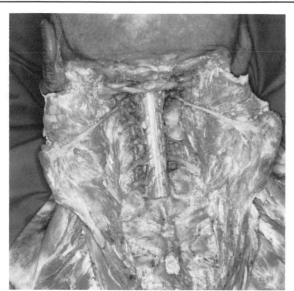
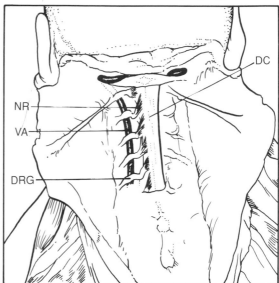

Figure 2–6. Dura and arachnoid have been removed from the spinal cord, exposing the root attachments and gross morphology of the posterior aspect of the spinal cord. The dorsal columns can be clearly seen. The arch of the atlas has been left in place for reference. DC, dorsal columns of spinal cord; DRG, dorsal root ganglion; NR, nerve rootlets; VA, vertebral artery.

stiffness to the spinal cord. When these attachments are severed, the spinal cord lengthens by at least 10 per cent because of its own weight.[5] After this initial lengthening, the spinal cord strongly resists elongation when further tensile forces are applied.

Axial compression forces applied to the spinal cord result initially in deformation and then buckling of the cord. The combined mechanical behavior of the spinal cord as a result of elongation and compression is much like the folding and unfolding of an accordion.[94]

When the dura mater with its closely associated arachnoid layer is removed from the spinal cord, the morphology of the spinal cord and the attachments of the nerve roots to the cord become evident (Fig. 2–6). The prominent posterior columns of the spinal cord with the midline posterior median septum can easily be seen in the cervical region. These important columns convey information concerning touch, pressure, sense of position, and movement toward the brain stem. The axons within these columns also convey information regarding two-point discrimination

and vibration. The posterior columns are especially abundant with axons derived from the joint receptors and muscle spindles. The anatomical relationship between the posterior columns of the spinal cord and the posterior wall of the spinal canal is instructive because it helps to explain several of the clinical signs and symptoms seen in myelopathy due to cervical spondylosis, such as hyperreflexia, proprioceptive dysfunction, difficulty in walking, paresthesias in the lower limbs, and clumsiness of the hands.

When the spinal cord is removed or pulled aside, the anterior aspect of the spinal canal can be examined (Fig. 2–7). The key anatomical structures are the posterior longitudinal ligament, intervertebral disc, vertebral body, and unciform joints (Fig. 2–8). Spondylitic changes in these elements can result in signs and symptoms of myelopathy because the anterior aspect of the spinal cord or the important anterior spinal artery is involved. Prolapse of the intervertebral disc, sequestered disc material, or bony spurs related to the unciform joints and vertebral body can mechanically compress the anterior aspect of

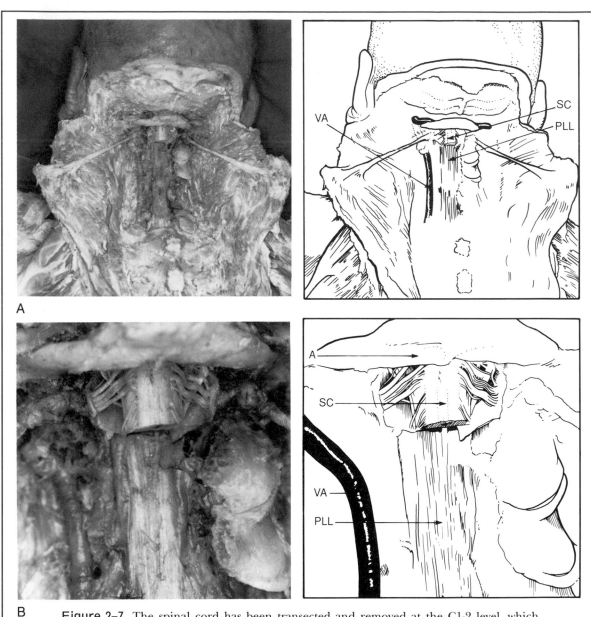

Figure 2–7. The spinal cord has been transected and removed at the C1-2 level, which exposes the posterior longitudinal ligament in both *A* and *B*. The C2-3 apophyseal joints are left in place in *B* for reference. In *B*, the closeup view allows the vertebral artery to be seen on the left and the nerve rootlets are seen attaching to the spinal cord. A, atlas; PLL, posterior longitudinal ligament; SC, transected spinal cord; VA, vertebral artery.

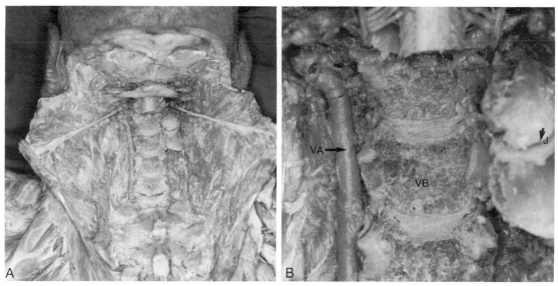

Figure 2–8. In *A*, the complete extent of the posterior longitudinal ligament has been removed, exposing the posterior aspect of the intervertebral disks and the vertebral bodies. In *B*, the closeup view allows for the laterally placed unciform joints and their relation to the apophyseal joints to be seen. VA, vertebral artery; VB, vertebral body; J, apophyseal joint.

the cord and related vasculature. Anteriorly placed spinal cord tracts potentially affected include the lateral spinothalamic, anterior spinothalamic, anterior spinocerebellar, and lateral corticospinal tracts.

The anterior wall of the spinal canal is a frequent site of bony intervertebral disc changes that occur as a result of spondylosis. Compromise of the vertebral canal size and compression of the spinal cord have been observed when the vertebral end plate develops spondylitic spurs and ridges. The sagittal diameter of the spinal canal decreases further when the cervical spine is extended or when the posterior longitudinal ligament is ossified.[27] Ossification of this ligament is a common cause of myelopathy in Oriental populations, but the condition is increasingly recognized in non-Oriental people.[22]

NERVE ROOT COMPLEX, SPINAL NERVE, AND RAMI

The nerve roots and their related structures are a multi-tissue complex composed of structur-

ally and neurophysiologically dissimilar elements.[27] The following elements are included in the complex:

1. Nerve root sleeves that house motor and sensory roots and their associated nerve rootlets. The sleeves are considered the theca and the roots are intrathecal structures

2. Highly vascularized and pressure-sensitive dorsal root ganglion, which in the spinal canal is still segregated from the motor root

3. Spinal nerve, which is formed when the ventral and dorsal roots merge

4. Vasculature of the nerve roots

Because of the dissimilarity of these neurophysiological elements, the term *nerve root complex* is a more appropriate and comprehensive term to use than *nerve root*, especially when discussing the pathophysiology of nerve root dysfunction. Pressure exerted on the root complex may trigger different neurodysfunctional phenomena, depending on which of the components is compromised.

The dorsal and ventral nerve roots attach to the spinal cord by way of a series of nerve rootlets

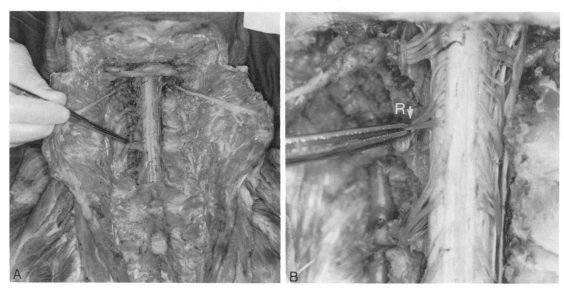

Figure 2–9. Attachment of the nerve roots to the spinal cord occurs by way of nerve rootlets. *A,* The probe is under the region where the ventral and dorsal rootlets form the roots, and then the two roots immediately unite to form the spinal nerve. Note the relation of the vertebral artery immediately anterior to the root complex. *B,* The probe is moving the dorsal rootlets aside to expose the more deeply placed ventral rootlets. The rootlets and roots are contained within the dural sheath.

(Fig. 2–9). These rootlets are slender and vary in number at different cervical levels. For example, the number of ventral rootlets in each spinal cord segment in the upper cervical spine is less than the number of rootlets per segment in the lower cervical spine. Because the ventral rootlets largely contain axons from motor neurons in the ventral horn of the spinal cord, more axons and therefore more rootlets would naturally be present in the regions of the cervical cord related to innervation of the upper extremity.

The series of dorsal and ventral rootlets related

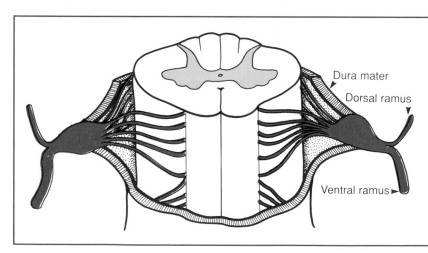

Figure 2–10. Formation of the nerve roots, spinal nerve, and rami.

Dura mater

Dorsal ramus

Ventral ramus

to each spinal cord segment converge to form the dorsal and ventral nerve roots, respectively. The dorsal root ganglion is related to the dorsal root because it contains the cell bodies that give rise to the axons forming the dorsal root. Axon cylinders leaving the dorsal root ganglion also travel toward the periphery. The nerve cell bodies related to the ventral root are located within the spinal cord itself.

The ventral root and dorsal root approach the cervical intervertebral foramen within the dural sheath. The dural sheath ends as a blind sac at approximately the region in which the two roots merge. The cervical spinal nerve is formed at approximately this region of the intervertebral foramen. This merger usually is immediately distal to the dorsal root ganglion at the region of the intervertebral foramen. At the lateral aspect of the intervertebral foramen, the spinal nerve branches to form the ventral and dorsal primary rami (Fig. 2–10).

Ventral rami of the cervical nerves contribute to the formation of the cervical plexus (ventral rami of the upper four cervical nerves) and brachial plexus (ventral rami of C5-T1). The cervical plexus supplies cutaneous nerves to the ventral and lateral aspects of the head and neck. The cutaneous nerves branching from the cervical plexus include the lesser occipital, great auricular, transverse colli, and supraclavicular nerves (Fig. 2–11). The muscular branches of the cervical plexus supply the deep cervical muscles of the spinal column, the hyoid muscles, and the diaphragm (Table 2–1). The ventral rami of the fifth cervical through the first thoracic segments form

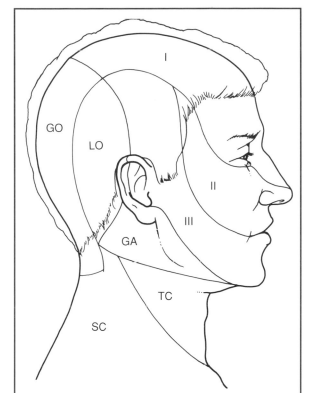

Figure 2–11. Sensory innervation of the head and neck. The trigeminal nerve supplies sensory innervation to the anterior face, the cervical plexus supplies the anterior and lateral head and neck, and the posterior ramus supplies the posterior head and neck. GA, greater auricular nerve; GO, greater occipital nerve; LO, lesser occipital nerve; SC, supraclavicular nerves; TC, transverse colli nerves; I, ophthalmic division of cranial nerve V; II, maxillary division of cranial nerve V; III, mandibular division of cranial nerve V.

Brachial Plexus C5-T1

the brachial plexus, which supplies motor and sensory innervation to the upper extremities.

The dorsal rami of the cervical nerves innervate the skin over the posterior aspect of the head and neck, deep muscles of the neck, and apophyseal joints and related ligaments and fascia. The suboccipital nerve, which is the dorsal ramus of C1, enters the suboccipital triangle and provides motor innervation to the muscles bordering this triangle: the rectus capitis posterior major and minor, superior oblique, and inferior oblique.

The largest of the dorsal rami of the cervical

Table 2–1. Muscular Branches of the Cervical Plexus *C1-4*
Rectus capitis anterior and lateralis
Longus capitis and colli
Geniohyoid
Thyrohyoid
Omohyoid
Sternohyoid
Sternothyroid
Diaphragm
Sternocleidomastoid
Trapezius
Levator scapulae
Scalenus medius

spinal nerves is from the second cervical spinal nerve (C2). It courses under the inferior oblique muscle and divides into a large medial branch known as the greater occipital nerve and a much smaller lateral branch. The greater occipital nerve pierces the semispinalis capitis (which it supplies) and trapezius muscles to become the cutaneous nerve supply to the posterior aspect and top of the occiput. Figure 2–6 shows this large nerve piercing the reflected muscles, and Figure 2–11 outlines its cutaneous distribution.

COURSE OF THE NERVE ROOT COMPLEX

With this understanding of the gross morphology of the nerve root complex, spinal nerve, and cervical rami, it is beneficial to further detail the path that the nerve root and spinal nerve follow to exit the spinal canal because this pathway has significant clinical relevance. Nerve roots exit the cervical intervertebral foramen by traveling over an extended bony channel located on top of the pedicle and transverse process of the cervical vertebrae. The anteromedial wall of this intervertebral foramen is formed by the uncovertebral joints, and the posterolateral wall is formed by the apophyseal joints. Spinal nerves related to the cervical spine exit above their corresponding vertebrae, with the first cervical spinal nerve (C1) exiting above the first cervical vertebrae, the second cervical spinal nerve (C2) exiting above the second cervical vertebrae, and so on. The eighth cervical spinal nerve (C8) exits between the seventh cervical and first thoracic vertebrae.

Cervical spondylosis, which results in structural alterations between the cervical articulations, can compromise nerve root function by mechanical compression to the axon cylinders themselves or to the nerve cell bodies of the dorsal root ganglion or by interference with the mechanisms of nerve root nutrition (described below). This condition can lead to cervical radicular signs or symptoms. In degenerative conditions such as spondylosis and uncovertebral joint arthrosis, the uncinate process becomes sclerotic and hypertrophic and the bone spurs often curve posteriorly. These spurs can result in fixation and compression of the nerve root bundle, which further compromises nerve root function.[27]

In their long course through the nerve root canal, the nerve root sleeve, dorsal root ganglion, and spinal nerve cannot yield superiorly because the root complex lies in a deep oblique furrow at the anterior aspect of the superior articular process.[27] This narrow furrow adjacent to the superior articular process places the nerve root complex immediately posterior to the vertebral artery (see Fig. 2–9). The cervical spinal nerves finally exit this extended nerve root canal through musculotendinous slits between the scalenus medius muscle and tendons, which are inserting into the tubercles of the transverse process.

NERVE ROOT COMPLEX DYSFUNCTION

The dorsal nerve roots consist primarily of axon cylinders whose nerve cell bodies are located in the dorsal root ganglion. The axon cylinders that travel peripherally from the dorsal root ganglion supply the cutaneous, joint, and muscle receptors in the periphery. The central projections from the dorsal root ganglion then enter the dorsal horn of the spinal cord by way of the dorsal rootlets.

The ventral rootlets are a series of axon cylinders that are extensions of nerve cell bodies located in the ventral horn of the spinal cord. These rootlets merge to form the ventral roots. Axons from these cell bodies (alpha motor neurons) innervate extrafusal muscle fibers and other axons (gamma motor neurons) supply the muscle spindles.

Because axons of the dorsal and ventral roots are extensions of nerve cell bodies, their survival and overall function are dependent on neuron cell body health. Interference with axonal transport mechanisms from the nerve cell body to the peripheral ends of the axon cylinder ultimately can alter the structure and function of the axon. Axons not only are responsible for conducting electrical impulses, but also serve as the transportation conduit for proteins and other essential substances synthesized in the nerve cell body.[29]

Mechanical deformation of normal, healthy spinal nerve roots typically leads to motor or sensory symptoms but not pain.[24] When the nerve root is subject to an inflammatory process, however, its mechanosensitivity increases and the characteristic symptoms of radicular pain can result when the nerve root is subject to compres-

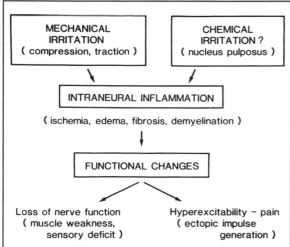

Figure 2–12. Mechanical and biochemical factors that cause nerve root pathology. (From Rydevik B, Garfin S: Spinal nerve root compression. *In* Szabo RM (ed): Nerve Compression Syndromes—Diagnosis and Treatment. Thorofare, NJ, Charles B. Slack, 1989.)

sion or tension. Thus, there is a fundamental difference between a healthy and an unhealthy nerve root in regard to its response to mechanical stresses (Fig. 2–12). A combination of mechanical stresses to the nerve root complex and an associated inflammatory process of the nerve root results in radicular pain.

Several mechanisms have been proposed as factors that contribute to the inflammatory process of the nerve root. A discrete intraneural circulation in combination with the diffusion of nutrients from the cerebrospinal fluid is responsible for maintenance of the health of the nerve roots.[25] Excessive tensile or compressive stresses may interfere with the normal function of the nerve roots by disrupting the availability of nutrients to maintain nerve root health, especially those that percolate from the cerebrospinal fluid. The development of an inflammatory exudate surrounding the nerve root or the subsequent establishment of perineural or intraneural fibrosis of the nerve root further compromises the movement of nutrients across the axon membrane. In addition to compressive or tensile stresses, altered nutrient diffusion within the nerve root renders it hypoxic and ischemic and potentially furthers neural fibrosis.

Several additional mechanisms have been proposed in regard to the cause of the inflamed or irritated nerve root. Degenerating disk material may produce an acidic environment that promotes adhesions around the nerve root and its dural sheath.[23] Autoimmune reactions caused by proteins leaking from the sequestered nucleus pulposus into the spinal canal have also been suggested as initiating the inflammatory tissue reactions seen surrounding degenerating discs and inflamed nerve roots.[4, 13] Thus it is clear that it is not solely mechanical stresses to the nerve root complex that result in radicular symptoms, but biochemical changes as well.

DORSAL ROOT GANGLION

The dorsal root ganglion, serving as the location of the nerve cell bodies, is even more vulnerable to mechanical stresses and biochemical changes than the axon cylinders of the nerve root. Two of the features of the dorsal root ganglion are its extensive microvascular network and tight capsule.[1] Mechanical compression to the ganglion is more critical than that to the root because it results in intraneural edema, increased tissue fluid pressure, and a decrease in nerve cell body blood supply within the ganglion. There is good evidence that mechanical compression of the healthy dorsal root ganglion, in contrast to compression on the normal nerve root, can initiate radiating pain.[29] Because the cells of the dorsal root ganglion maintain the viability of the centrally and peripherally projecting axons through axoplasmic transport, spontaneous discharge of the axons caused by biochemical or biomechanical stress to their parent nerve cell bodies may result in aberrant afferent input into the central nervous system.[8] Because head and face symptoms often are associated with neck disorders, it is important to note that the neurons associated with the trigeminal ganglion, which are largely responsible for sensory innervation to the face and are functionally similar to the dorsal root ganglion, have a lesser capacity for such spontaneous discharges.[7]

The dorsal root ganglion is mechanosensitive and produces several important neuropeptides important for pain modulation.[32, 33] Although substance P and somatostatin are the best known

Table 2–2. Neuropeptides of the Dorsal Root Ganglion

Substance P
Somatostatin
Vasoactive intestinal polypeptide
Gastrin-releasing peptide
Calcitonin gene-related peptide
Dynorphin
Enkephalin
Galanin
Neurotensin
Angiotensin II
Cholecystokinin

neuropeptides related to the dorsal root ganglion, they are only two of several neuropeptides synthesized within the dorsal root ganglia cell bodies and delivered by axonal transport to the central processes (axon terminals in the spinal cord) and peripheral processes (axon terminals in the innervated tissues) (Table 2–2). These neuropeptides are important in the mediation of pain as well as in the mediation of the inflammatory response. Because an understanding of the inflammatory response is essential to the management of mechanical neck disorders, the relevance of this response to neural influences is briefly discussed.

MEDIATION OF THE INFLAMMATORY RESPONSE

The primary modes of mediation for the inflammatory response are non-neurogenic and neurogenic. Although the modes are different, it is important to appreciate both because they are responsible for the sensitization of peripheral nerve endings that occurs as a result of tissue injury. This sensitization process contributes to the initiation of afferent impulses toward the dorsal root ganglion and, ultimately, the central nervous system.

When the cell walls of tissue have been injured or disrupted, several chemical mediators are released. The chemical mediators of pain released from non-neural tissues (non-neurogenic mediation) include bradykinin, serotonin, histamine, and acetylcholine.[18] These non-neurogenic chemicals mediate the pain response by activating the afferent free nerve endings associated with nociceptive nerve endings and increase the sensitivity to pain by lowering the activation threshold of the nociceptive terminal.

Arachidonic acid is released from the injured cell walls and is acted on by two distinct enzyme systems, which results in the production of pros-

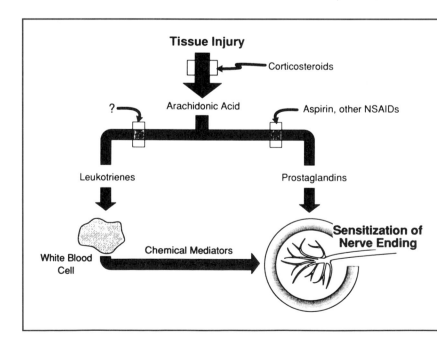

Figure 2–13. Effect of tissue injury on the sensitization process of the nerve ending. (Adapted from Weinstein J: Neurophysiology of pain. *In* Mayer T, Mooney V, Gatchel R (eds): Contemporary Conservative Care for Painful Spinal Disorders. Philadelphia, Lea & Febiger, 1991.)

taglandins and leukotrienes. The particular enzyme responsible for the conversion of arachidonic acid to prostaglandin is cyclooxygenase. It is this enzyme action that aspirin and other nonsteroidal anti-inflammatory medications appear to block (Fig. 2–13). Leukotrienes are an important product in this biochemical sequence because they are chemical mediators that lower the threshold response of the nociceptors. Leukotrienes also mediate the influx of white blood cells to an area of injury. They do not appear to be suppressed by nonsteroidal anti-inflammatory medications.

In contrast to non-neural mediation, neurogenic mediators of pain, referred to as neuropeptides, are produced within the nerve cell bodies of the dorsal root ganglion. Neuropeptides course peripherally toward the distal receptors in injured tissue as well as centrally toward the spinal cord by way of axoplasmic transport. Neuropeptides that travel distally through the axon cylinders to be released at the site of injured tissues have a pronounced influence on the inflammatory process.[26] They can stimulate increased blood flow, influence vascular permeability at the injured tissue site, and facilitate the release of histamine from mast cells. They also stimulate the release of leukotrienes from mast cells, which attract white blood cells to the area of tissue disturbance.[26] These factors contribute to a state of hyperalgesia of injured tissue, which increases the mechanosensitivity of the afferent nerve endings and potentiates the inflammatory response.

Neuropeptides are also transported peripherally to the dorsal horn of the spinal cord, which serves as the first synapse for the pain pathway and, thus, is the initial location for neural synapses involved with pain modulation. Neurogenic mediators such as substance P reach the second-order neurons involved in the pain pathways that provide information destined to upper levels of the central nervous system. Although substance P has been the neuropeptide most extensively studied, many others are known to be used by pain afferent fibers to communicate within the central nervous system.

The peripheral sensitization caused by non-neurogenic and neurogenic influences also results in central sensitization. As the hypersensitized receptors in the periphery flood the central nervous system with afferent pain transmission, changes in the sensitivity of the second-order neuron (the neuron or neurons that the axons from the dorsal root ganglion synapse with in the spinal cord) also occur. The synaptic membrane of the second-order neuron is altered when a continuous cascade of afferent pain impulses reaches it. Thus, intensely painful conditions can result in hypersensitization of the central nervous system because this is the location of the second-order neurons. This sequence of events provides the rationale for the use of local and topical anesthetics in areas of intense pain. By minimizing the peripheral pain response, the central nervous system's response is lessened.

Neurogenic and non-neurogenic mediators of pain play key roles in influencing the chemical milieu of the central nervous system and the site of tissue injury and have especially important functions in the propagation of the inflammatory response. The interplay between inflammation, the nervous system, and, ultimately, the subjective experience of pain is unique.

CLINICAL CORRELATES OF NERVE ROOT, RAMUS, AND NERVE DYSFUNCTION

Dysfunction of the neural structures is a common sequelae of many cervical spine disorders. Because the structure of the nerve root and spinal nerves, the influence the inflammatory process has on neural tissue, and the influence the nervous system has on the inflammatory process itself have been addressed, individual segmental nerve root and nerve dysfunction patterns resulting in clinical signs and symptoms can now be described.

The C2 nerve root complex is difficult to definitively assess. Compression or irritation of the C2 nerve root is surmised to result in unilateral pain or paresthesias in the upper neck, suboccipital region, and area surrounding the mastoid process. Occipital hypalgesia is also a possibility.

The dorsal ramus of C2 serves as an afferent pain pathway from the atlantoaxial apophyseal joint articulation. The greater occipital nerve, which is the large medial branch of the C2 dorsal ramus, is thought to be vulnerable to entrapment as it pierces the semispinalis capitis muscle and nuchal fascia in its course toward the occiput. Tenderness over the posterior and cranial aspects of the occiput may occur as a result of such entrapment.

The C3 and C4 nerve roots are difficult to assess with muscle tests or reflexes because of the inability to isolate specific muscles innervated by these roots. The pain pattern resulting from irritation of these roots is considered to be over the lateral aspect of the neck, reaching as far inferiorly as the acromioclavicular joint.

The C5 nerve root pain pattern reaches into the shoulder and upper arm, with paresthesias extending toward the distal arm and proximal forearm. Muscles innervated by the C5 nerve root that may show weakness on clinical examination include the deltoid, supraspinatus, infraspinatus, and elbow flexors. The reflex most often affected is the biceps.

The C6 nerve root pain pattern extends into the anterior aspect of the arm down to the elbow, and complaints of paresthesias on the radial side of the forearm and into the thumb are common. The elbow flexors and radial wrist extensors are weakened, and the brachioradialis reflex is altered.

The C7 nerve root pain pattern radiates down the posterior forearm and often features paresthesias in the index, long, and ring fingers. The triceps muscle and occasionally the wrist extensors and flexors are weakened. The triceps reflex is an important assessment of C7 nerve root function.

Compression or irritation of the C8 nerve root causes pain in the interscapular region that radiates into the medial aspect of the arm, often accompanied by paresthesias along the ulnar border of the forearm. Muscles weakened with a C8 nerve root lesion include the flexor carpi ulnaris, flexor digitorum profundus, and intrinsic muscles of the hand.

Lesions of the T1 nerve root may produce weakness of intrinsic hand muscles as well as ptosis, miosis, or anhydrosis of the eye because the first thoracic segment is part of the outflow from the sympathetic portion of the autonomic nervous system. T1 nerve root lesions are less common but are mentioned here because the nerve root pain pattern into the axilla and medial aspect of the upper arm mimics the pain of Pancoast tumors. These neoplasms arise in the apical parietal pleura and constitute 5 per cent of all bronchogenic tumors.[30] The tumor may invade the stellate ganglion of the sympathetic chain, leading to Horner's syndrome (described below), as well as the brachial plexus. Pain in this region should be carefully evaluated because neoplasms need to be considered in the differential diagnosis.

The signs and symptoms that differentiate nerve root lesions from peripheral nerve lesions need to be carefully assessed. In general, sensory symptoms that occur as a result of cervical nerve root compression or irritation follow a dermatomal distribution, but anesthesia is rare because of dermatome overlap. Sensory disturbances from peripheral nerve lesions are more clearly demarcated and often have an accompanying motor deficit. Although pain is a primary complaint with nerve root involvement, a specific sensory deficit is not typically noted. Symptoms from peripheral nerve lesions usually are not altered with head and neck movements, coughing, or sneezing, whereas these maneuvers aggravate the pain from nerve root involvement.

As noted above in the discussion of individual nerve roots, radicular symptoms are characterized by proximal pain and distal paresthesias, and this is an important aspect to clarify during the examination. Finally, pain from an irritated lower cervical nerve root occasionally can be relieved by resting the arm in an abducted position—for example, by placing the hand on the head to keep the arm elevated.[2] This maneuver is thought to decrease tension on the nerve root and therefore alter nerve root symptoms. This invites further discussion on the concept of neural tension tests.

NEURAL TENSION TESTS

The clinician often is required to differentiate between intrinsic shoulder pain and the shoulder pain stemming from cervical spine involvement. One of the means to provide information in regard to the status of neural tissues associated with the cervical spine and brachial plexus is through the use of neural tension tests. Although the clinical application of neural tension tests is discussed in Chapter 5, it is germane to a discussion of nerve root dysfunction to examine the theory and biomechanics of these tests at this point. To understand the rationale behind neural tension testing, one must distinguish between compressive and tensile forces placed on the nerve root complex.

Compression tests are fairly well understood. The purpose of the tests is to reduce the lumen of the intervertebral foramen by way of compression of the cervical spine or by combined movements such as extension, lateral flexion, and rotation. If the nerve root complex is irritated or inflamed, it is mechanically sensitive to this compressive force and pain can be provoked along a dermatomal distribution. One of the limitations of cervical spine tests is that many patients with neck pain have difficulty assuming these combined positions because of the muscle guarding associated with their syndrome.

To supplement these compression tests, clinicians have endeavored to implement neural tension tests for the upper extremities and neck that could serve as analogs for the straight-leg–raise test (a type of neural tension assessment) for the low back. The straight-leg raise, using various degrees of hip flexion, adduction, internal rotation, knee extension, and ankle dorsiflexion, places a tensile force through the sciatic nerve and its terminating branches as well as the lumbosacral plexus.

Neural tension tests for the upper extremities might be indicated in the following situations:

1. When arm or hand symptoms cannot be reproduced with examination of cervical or upper-extremity joint and soft tissue assessment
2. Chronic upper quarter conditions
3. Postsurgical conditions of the upper quarter
4. Habitual shoulder girdle elevation, especially with shoulder movements
5. Increase in upper-quarter pain with cervical

rotation and lateral bending away from the side of pain

Elvey was one of the first to describe tests for the upper extremities that could selectively stress the cervical nerve roots.[12] One of the limitations to the neural tension tests of the upper extremities appeared to be the relative fixation of the nerve roots by way of the tent-like arrangement of the dura mater at the cervical intervertebral foramen and the fibrous tethering of the nerve root as it courses along its extensive bony channel over the pedicles and transverse processes. Elvey was able to demonstrate on cadaver specimens, however, that although nerve root motion was restricted, movement of the arm elicited motion and tension on the cervical nerve roots, especially at the C5, C6, and C7 levels. No effect was observed at the C8 and T1 levels.[12]

Using the principles developed for straight-leg–raise testing, combined positions of the upper quarter, including the cervical spine, shoulder girdle, glenohumeral, elbow, forearm, wrist, and hand, have been suggested as a means to place a tensile stress through the peripheral nerves, brachial plexus, and, ultimately, nerve root complex of the upper extremity and cervical spine. Table 2–3 lists upper-quarter positions that increase tension of the brachial plexus and cervical nerve roots by way of the median and ulnar nerves.

The course of the median nerve on the ventral side of the elbow and of the ulnar nerve on the dorsal aspect illustrate the difference in tension developed based on whether the elbow is extended or flexed. In practical terms, the positioning used for the median nerve is of more clinical value because the limited movement of the C8 and T1 nerve roots and the additional tethering

Table 2–3. Neural Tension Tests	
Median Nerve Bias	**Ulnar Nerve Bias**
Shoulder girdle depression	Shoulder girdle depression
Shoulder abduction (110 degrees)	Shoulder abduction (100 degrees)
Shoulder external rotation	Shoulder external rotation
Forearm supinated	Forearm supinated
Wrist and fingers extended	Wrist extended
Elbow extended	Elbow flexed
Neck laterally fixed	Neck laterally flexed

of the ulnar nerve behind the medial epicondyle make the ulnar nerve tension test less sensitive. The most practical way to administer the more sensitive median nerve test is to preset the shoulder girdle, wrist, and hand and then carefully and slowly move the elbow toward extension to assess the response. The responses elicited include reproduction of the patient's complaint, an asymmetry of elbow or wrist position when two sides are compared, and symptoms that can be altered with neck position.

Therefore, as with the straight-leg raise, test results focus on motion limitation in the extremity and the pain pattern induced by testing. The most useful way to assess limitation of motion is to note if there is a limitation of passive elbow extension because of pain or where during the excursion of elbow extension pain begins. The pain pattern should follow those rules known for root irritation (i.e., peripheralizing symptoms along a dermatome). Pain or altered sensation in the C5 and C6 dermatomes and to a lesser extent in the C7 dermatome is the most common. Tension on the nerve root complex can be further increased by contralateral lateral flexion and by sidegliding of the cervical spine while the upper-extremity position is maintained. Such testing procedures are also valuable in ruling out pain of shoulder origin.

SYMPATHETIC NERVOUS SYSTEM

Clinicians who deal with cervical spine disorders should have a working understanding of the autonomic nervous system, specifically the sympathetic component. An understanding of the sympathetic nervous system is relevant to a discussion of cervical spine disorders for two primary reasons.

1. The sympathetic chain ganglion, which lies within the carotid sheath, courses along the anterolateral aspect of the neck and, thus, has the potential to be injured with trauma, such as that which might occur with acceleration injuries, like any other soft tissues of the neck.

2. Increased activation of the sympathetic nervous system affects a person's perception of pain and response to painful stimuli through its strong influence on the person's emotional state.

As a result, the sympathetic nervous system plays an important role in painful states of the head and neck caused by mechanical injury to the sympathetic chain or by way of neuropsychological and neuroendocrine influences.

The primary components of the autonomic nervous system are the parasympathetic, sympathetic, and enteric systems. The enteric system is largely concerned with autonomic innervation to the abdominal viscera and is not considered in this text. Only the parasympathetic and sympathetic nervous systems are discussed here, with the primary consideration given to the sympathetic system.

Cell bodies that give rise to axons that contribute to the parasympathetic nervous system are largely centered in the brain stem and sacral spinal cord (craniosacral outflow) and are known as preganglionic neurons (Fig. 2–14). Cell bodies that give rise to axons that contribute to the sympathetic nervous system largely originate in the intermediolateral cell column of the thoracic and upper lumbar spinal cord (thoracolumbar outflow) and are also referred to as preganglionic neurons. Despite the limited origins of both systems, nearly all smooth muscle, cardiac muscle, and glands have parasympathetic and sympathetic innervation through unique branching and synapsing patterns (Fig. 2–15). The viscera also provide afferent information to the central nervous system, which is a component of autonomic nervous system function; hence, the autonomic nervous system is concerned with both visceral efferent and visceral afferent function.

A key component of the sympathetic system relevant to neck disorders is the sympathetic chain ganglia. Because the origin of the sympathetic preganglionic neurons is the thoracic and upper lumbar spinal cord, the neurons must use the sympathetic chain to extend upward to reach target organs in the cervical spine, upper extremities, head, and face (see Fig. 2–14). The preganglionic neurons that exit from the thoracic and lumbar spinal cord enter the sympathetic chain, which is located immediately adjacent to the spine, and have several synaptic options within the chain:

1. They can synapse with a second neuron in the sympathetic chain at the same level at which they exit the spinal cord. The axon of the second neuron ascends the sympathetic chain and then leaves the chain to reach its target organ.

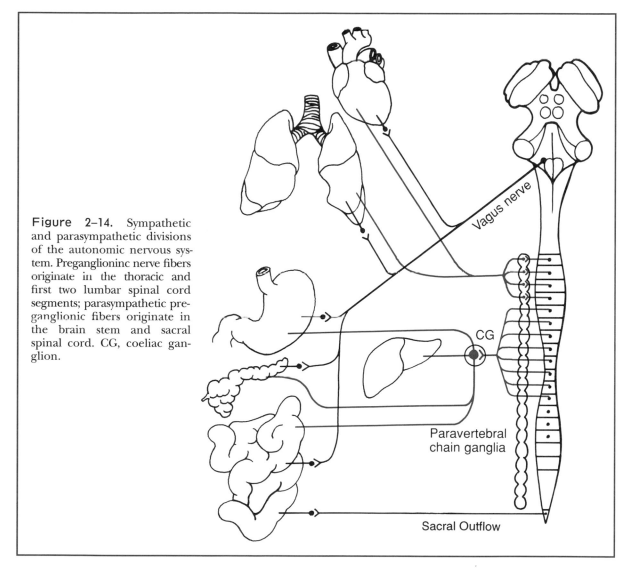

Figure 2–14. Sympathetic and parasympathetic divisions of the autonomic nervous system. Preganglioninc nerve fibers originate in the thoracic and first two lumbar spinal cord segments; parasympathetic preganglionic fibers originate in the brain stem and sacral spinal cord. CG, coeliac ganglion.

2. They can exit the spinal cord, enter the sympathetic chain at the same level, and travel up the sympathetic chain to reach the cervical sympathetic ganglia, whereupon they synapse with a second neuron. The second neuron then leaves the chain to reach its target organ.

3. They can exit the spinal cord, enter the sympathetic chain at the same level, travel up the chain, and pass through it to reach the target organ. On the target organ, they synapse with a second neuron.

Regardless of the option, a synapse with a post-ganglionic neuron occurs either within the sympathetic chain or on the target organ.

The key sympathetic chain ganglia related to the head and neck in which these synapses occur are the stellate, middle cervical, and superior cervical ganglia (Fig. 2–16). Most postganglionic neurons (the second neuron of the synaptic sequence) destined for the head and face then leave these ganglia and travel along branches of the carotid arteries toward their target organs in the neck, head, and face.

The vertebral artery also carries sympathetic

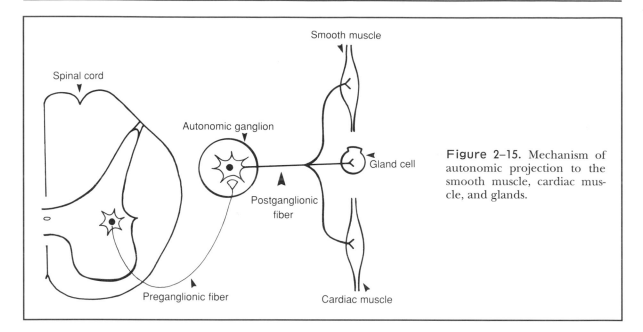

Figure 2–15. Mechanism of autonomic projection to the smooth muscle, cardiac muscle, and glands.

nerve fibers on its surface in its course through the transverse foramen of the cervical vertebrae.[35] These autonomic fibers not only supply the smooth muscle of the blood vessels, but also provide filaments that contribute to the sinuvertebral nerve, which innervates structures within the spinal canal, including the posterior longitudinal ligament and the intervertebral disk. Postganglionic nerve fibers from the sympathetic chain also accompany the ventral rami, dorsal rami, and sinuvertebral nerve to their various destinies in the upper extremities, cervical tissues, and spinal canal.

One of the more severe cervical problems related to stretch injury or hemorrhage to the sympathetic chain is the Barré syndrome.[3] This syndrome features suboccipital headaches, vertigo, tinnitus, dysesthesias of the hands provoked by stress or emotional disruption, and craniofacial complaints such as pain, numbness, and nausea. The injury may be to the sympathetic chain ganglia itself or to the ventral roots from C5-T1, which carry sympathetic nerve fibers into the upper extremities.[21]

Sympathetic nerve fibers from the superior cervical ganglion innervate the dilator pupillary muscle and the smooth muscle that helps to elevate the eyelid. Horner's syndrome, a condition that results in a constricted pupil (miosis) and a drooping eyelid (ptosis), can occur as a result of injury to the sympathetic chain ganglia in the neck, such as that following acceleration injury, and should be carefully evaluated in an inspection of the head and neck.

Several features of the sympathetic nervous system deserve mention. One is the ratio of preganglionic nerve fibers to postganglionic nerve fibers. In the sympathetic nervous system, this ratio is about 1:10, whereas in the parasympathetic nervous system, the ratio is about 1:3. Therefore, sympathetic reactions are more widespread and diffuse, and a small stimulus has the potential for a broader response.

Another difference is in the type of neurotransmitter released at the terminals of the postganglionic neuron. In the sympathetic system, norepinephrine, a catecholamine, is released, whereas in the parasympathetic system, the neurotransmitter is acetylcholine. The effects of sympathetic system activation is longer lasting because the action of norepinephrine is terminated by reuptake of the transmitter by the nerve terminal. In addition, norepinephrine that escapes reuptake enters the circulation, further spreading sympathetic effects. By contrast, acetylcholine action is more rapidly terminated by enzyme activity. Thus, not only are sympathetic actions more widespread because of this diffuse distribution of the catecholamines, but they are also more enduring.

Another feature of the sympathetic nervous system is the direct innervation of the adrenal medulla by sympathetic nervous system preganglionic nerve fibers. When the adrenal medulla is stimulated by these preganglionic neurons, epinephrine is released, which causes a generalized body reaction due to this circulating catecholamine. Widespread reactions include elevated blood pressure and pulse rate and such emotions as fear and anger.

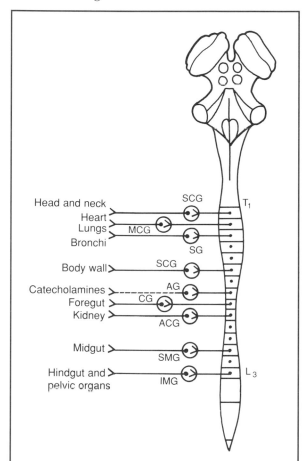

Figure 2-16. Sympathetic chain ganglia and their relations to their respective target organs. AG, adrenal gland; ACG, aorticorenal ganglion; CG, coeliac ganglion; IMG, inferior mesenteric ganglion; MCG, middle cervical ganglion; SCG, superior cervical ganglion; SG, stellate ganglion; SMG, superior mesenteric ganglion.

Control of the autonomic nervous system from higher levels is by way of a highly complex circuitry. Key structures include the hypothalamus and locus ceruleus and regions of the limbic system. Most areas of the brain act indirectly on the autonomic nervous system by way of the hypothalamus. The hypothalamus can act on the neurons of the brain stem that control parasympathetic function and the neurons in the thoracic and lumbar spinal cord by controlling sympathetic function through descending tracts. The hypothalamus also directly influences the autonomic nervous system through the release of hormones, which bathe the autonomic ganglia and thereby propagate visceral responses.

Although the hypothalamus is considered an important regulator of autonomic nervous system function, the locus ceruleus—a cluster of cell bodies in the pons of the brain stem—has been demonstrated to synthesize, store, and release norepinephrine. It is considered to have the highest density of norepinephrine of any cluster of neurons in the brain.[9] This nucleus distributes nerve fibers throughout the central nervous system and is regarded as the principal source of norepinephrine in the central nervous system.[10] The locus ceruleus may be one of the most important regions of the nervous system concerned with the modulation of psychological stress, emotional distress, adverse immune reactions, and generalized sympathetic-parasympathetic imbalance.[19]

Although the clinician is continually searching for the mechanical basis of a neck disorder, the influence of the sympathetic nervous system on the painful state should be kept in mind. Because pain is an emotional experience rather than a primary sensory one, those systems that contribute to the regulation of emotion factor heavily into the perception of pain. Stressors in a person's life, which can profoundly affect sympathetic nervous system activity, influence the perception of pain primarily because of the neurochemical changes they evoke.

TRIGEMINAL NERVE SYSTEM

Mechanical disorders of the neck frequently are accompanied by symptoms in the head, face, or temporomandibular region. In addition, it is common for temporomandibular joint involvement or soft tissue injuries related to the face and head to refer pain to the cervical spine. Because the trigeminal nerve system is largely responsible for the sensory innervation of the face and temporomandibular regions and because cervical spine disorders often present with head and face symptoms, it is essential that the clinician have a working knowledge of this system.

The trigeminal nerve system provides motor innervation to several muscles by way of three major branches: the ophthalmic, maxillary, and mandibular. The ophthalmic and maxillary branches are primarily sensory nerves, whereas the mandibular branch is sensory to the face and provides motor innervation to the muscles of mastication. The distribution of the sensory nerves is shown in Figure 2–11.

Just as the dorsal root ganglion is the location of cell bodies for the sensory afferents related to the trunk and extremities, the trigeminal (or semilunar) ganglion is the location of cell bodies concerned with sensory afferent nerves to the face. This ganglion is located immediately outside the brain stem, just as the dorsal root ganglion is located immediately outside the spinal cord. Sensations such as pain and temperature are carried through this ganglion into the brain stem.

In contrast, proprioceptive input from the face and the sensation of touch are subserved using unique pathways. Instead of the trigeminal ganglion serving as cell bodies for nerve fibers supplying proprioceptive input, a cluster of cell bodies known as the mesencephalic nucleus (for proprioception) and the principal nucleus (for touch) are located within the brain stem itself (Fig. 2–17). Receptors such as muscle spindles and Golgi tendon organs and the various mechanoreceptors are supplied by these nuclei.

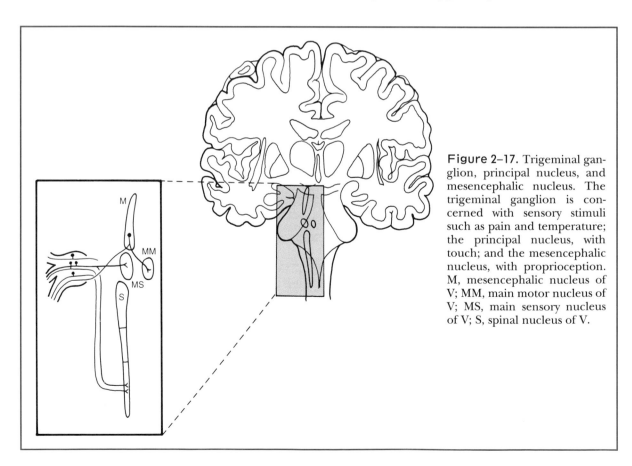

Figure 2–17. Trigeminal ganglion, principal nucleus, and mesencephalic nucleus. The trigeminal ganglion is concerned with sensory stimuli such as pain and temperature; the principal nucleus, with touch; and the mesencephalic nucleus, with proprioception. M, mesencephalic nucleus of V; MM, main motor nucleus of V; MS, main sensory nucleus of V; S, spinal nucleus of V.

A unique aspect of the pain and temperature afferent nerve fibers that arise from the trigeminal ganglion and enter the central nervous system is that these nerve fibers descend through the brain stem into the cervical spinal cord. In the lower brain stem and cervical spinal cord, these neurons synapse with a second neuron located in the spinal tract of the trigeminal. This second neuron then crosses the central nervous system to ascend toward the thalamus (see Fig. 2–17).

Trigeminal neuralgia is a severe onset of facial pain with an acute hypersensitivity to touch, usually in the distribution of one of the branches of the facial nerve. Symptoms usually include recurrent 10- to 30-second bouts of intense, sharp pain. The skin around the eyes and nose often serves as a trigger area for the paroxysms of pain. Sympathetic disturbances such as lacrimation and blanching of the skin on the involved side are common. The cause is unclear, although viral infection of the trigeminal ganglion or nerve, pressure on the nerve, and disturbances within the spinal tract of the trigeminal nerve and the brain stem have been implicated.[16] The clinician should recognize that the diagnosis ultimately is made from the history, description of pain, and dermatomal distribution of symptoms. Therefore, the response to medications and surgical or nonsurgical interventions rests with the patient's subjective response.

As mentioned earlier, the mandibular division of the trigeminal nerve has both motor and sensory functions. Besides a large cutaneous and mucous membrane region of innervation, the sensory division of the nerve is responsible for innervation to the temporomandibular joint. Pain from this joint can arise from any of the ligaments, joint capsule, and related connective tissue structures.

The motor division of the trigeminal nerve innervates the muscles of mastication, including the temporalis, masseter, pterygoid, mylohyoid, and digastric muscles. These muscles often are involved with myofascial syndromes associated with temporomandibular joint pain. Sustained contraction of these muscles results in such symptoms as muscle tenderness, bruxism, and abnormal disc mechanics potentially leading to internal derangement.[15] These aspects concerning sensory and motor functions of the mandibular division of the trigeminal nerve are important neural considerations in the evaluation of temporomandibular joint dysfunction.

INTERPLAY BETWEEN THE VESTIBULAR AND OCULAR SYSTEMS AND THE CERVICAL SPINE

This section is concerned with the neurophysiological rationale behind the signs and symptoms that occasionally accompany cervical spine disorders, such as balance disturbances and visual problems. A series of reflex connections exist between the motor neurons that innervate the muscles of the cervical spine, the vestibular apparatus, the auditory apparatus, and the motor neuron pools related to eye movements. This helps to explain several of the more disconcerting secondary problems associated with cervical spine injuries.

Even though the sense of balance is largely unconscious, it plays an essential role in coordinating head and neck posture and eye movements. Although the receptors for balance serve several other important roles within the nervous system, discussion here is limited to functional relations with the head and neck. It is beyond the scope of this chapter to present more than a clinical perspective, and the reader is referred to other sources for detailed neuroanatomy and neurophysiology.[6, 17]

It is important that the clinician understand the vestibular system and its associated reflexes because of the effect that acceleration and deceleration forces have on the inner ear, such as those that might occur with motor vehicle accidents. Such injuries can result in postural disorders and altered states of muscle tone in the cervical spine.[11]

The vestibular system is located in the vestibule of the inner ear and is composed of the two primary organs of equilibrium: the semicircular canals and the otoliths. Mechanical displacement of the head results in the conversion of this energy to a neural signal within these sense organs, which is then interpreted and acted on by different regions of the central nervous system.

The sensory receptors in the semicircular canals and the otoliths are sensitive to changes in the acceleration of the head, such as that which occurs with change of head position or speed of movement, and in the position of the head with respect to gravity. Because of their arrangement, these organs of equilibrium can detect head motion and position in any of the cardinal planes.

Afferent information coming from the semicircular canals and otoliths is relayed to the brain stem by the vestibular portion of the eighth cranial nerve. The eighth cranial nerve in turn transmits this information to a large cluster of nerve cells in the medulla known as the vestibular nucleus. The vestibular input is also directed into the cerebellum.

The connection with the vestibular nucleus is especially important because this nucleus gives rise to axons that form descending spinal cord tracts that influence head, neck, and trunk posture as well as to axons that connect with brain stem nuclei that control eye movement. The practical relevance of these connections is that the eyes can remain fixated on one point even though the head and neck are moving.

The vestibular nucleus is one of the largest complexes of nerve cell bodies in the brain stem. It is so extensive that it can be subdivided into four components: the lateral, medial, superior, and inferior vestibular nuclei. The clinical relevance of this nuclear complex is that distinct portions are responsible for important functions of the cervical spine, head, and eyes (Fig. 2–18).

The lateral and medial vestibular nuclei serve as examples of the interplay between motor activity and the vestibular apparatus. The lateral vestibular nucleus receives input from the vestibular apparatus as well as from the spinal cord and cerebellum. The output from this nucleus is then directed superiorly in the brain stem toward the motor nuclei of the ocular muscles and inferiorly toward the ventral horn cells and gamma motor neurons of the cervical spinal cord. The tract formed in the spinal cord, referred to as the lateral vestibulospinal tract, is an important motor tract that innervates alpha and gamma motor neurons related to muscles of the limbs.

The medial vestibular nucleus also receives input from the vestibular apparatus. This nucleus also sends neural connections to nuclei of the ocular muscles and gives rise to the medial vestibulospinal tract, which descends into the cervical region of the spinal cord. This descending tract is largely concerned with the innervation of the neck muscles and upper back muscles. This tract is largely responsible for the coordinated movements between the neck muscles and the eyes as a result of vestibular input. The medial vestibulospinal tract from one side of the brain stem projects bilaterally to the cervical spinal cord, and thus, one vestibular nucleus can influence cervical muscles on either or both sides of the spine. Furthermore, input from the muscle spindles of the neck muscles provides sensory input back to the medial vestibular nucleus, which allows for

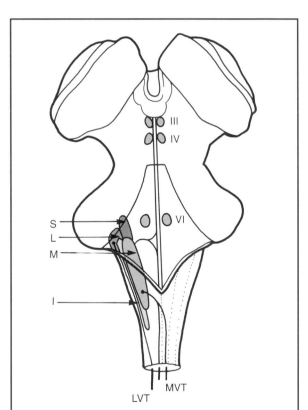

Figure 2–18. Vestibular nuclear complex. Located in the medulla, this nuclear complex gives rise to the vestibulospinal tracts and the connections to the motor neurons that control the extraocular muscles. I, inferior nucleus; L, lateral (Deiter's) nucleus; LVT, lateral vestibulospinal tract; M, medial nucleus; MVT, medial vestibulospinal tract; S, superior nucleus.

continual update of cervical spine proprioception to the nucleus.

The influence of the vestibular apparatus on the vestibulospinal tracts and, ultimately, the motor neurons responsible for innervation of muscles of the head and neck should be considered during the assessment of acceleration injuries. Oscillation forces of the head that occur as a result of a motor vehicle accident may cause inner ear dysfunction and a disorder of postural control. These postural control changes are reflected in abnormal muscle tension states in the antigravity muscles of the head and neck as well as in disorders of balance and equilibrium.[11]

Cervical, Ocular, and Vestibular Reflexes

Much of the coordination between the head, neck, eyes, and vestibular apparatus is reflexive rather than conscious effort. Vestibular reflexes that result in motor responses from the neck are termed vestibulocollic reflexes; vestibular reflexes that act on the limbs are vestibulospinal reflexes. Cervicocollic reflexes are those inputs from the muscle spindles of the neck muscles and receptors in the joints that cause neck muscle contraction. For example, turning the head stretches muscles that elicit muscle spindle activity, which results in the contraction of the same muscles.

Vestibulo-ocular reflexes are initiated by input from the vestibular apparatus and result in eye movement. An example of this is the observation that as the head is actively rotated, the extraocular muscles move the eyes at the precise velocity necessary to keep visual images fixed on the retina.[14] As you read this page, your head turns to the right while your eyes compensate by rotating toward the left, allowing you to keep the words of the page fixed and unblurred on the retina.

Visual input also initiates specific reflex movements of the head and neck. Input from the retinas provides information to several brain stem regions, one of which is a large cluster of cells in the midbrain known as the superior colliculus. An important descending motor tract that originates from the superior colliculus is the tectospinal tract. This tract innervates the motor neurons that innervate the ocular muscles as well as the motor neurons that supply the musculature of the head and neck. The main function of such an arrangement is to assure that head and neck motor activity is coordinated with eye movement.

The inability to position the head and neck to optimize the sense organs often is a source of frustration in patients with neck pain. Although the afferent input arrives at the appropriate brain stem region, it is difficult for the patient to initiate the appropriate motor response because of pain or dysfunction. For this reason, one of the prime treatment goals for patients with neck disorders is to restore painless, coordinated motion as rapidly as possible.

SUMMARY

The neurosciences of the cervical spine have a degree of complexity found in no other region of the axial skeleton. Many syndromes of the neck are not of a purely mechanical nature, but display evidence of neuromotor, neuroendocrine, and neuropsychological influences. This chapter provides an overview of the gross morphology and functional neuroanatomy of the central and peripheral nervous systems, which often are involved in cervical spine disorders. It is important to appreciate not only the role the nerve root plays in painful syndromes of the neck, but also the consequences of autonomic and motor control dysfunction.

REFERENCES

1. Arvidson B: Distribution of intravenously injected protein tracers in peripheral ganglia of adult mice. Exp Neurol 63:388–410, 1979.
2. Beatty RM, Fowler FD, Hanson EJ Jr: The abducted arm as a sign of ruptured cervical disc. Neurosurgery 21:731–732, 1987.
3. Bland JH: Disorders of the Cervical Spine. Philadelphia, WB Saunders, 1987, pp 224–225.
4. Bobechko WP, Hirsch C: Auto-immune response to nucleus pulposus in the rabbit. J Bone Joint Surg 47B:574–580, 1965.
5. Breig A: Biomechanics of the Central Nervous System: Some Basic Normal and Pathological Phenomena. Stockholm, Almquist & Wiksell, 1960.
6. Brodal A: Neurological Anatomy in Relation to Clinical

Medicine. 3rd ed. New York, Oxford University Press, 1981.

7. Burchiel KJ, Wyler AR, Harris AB: Epileptogenic agents applied to the trigeminal ganglia: Absence of neuro-hyperexcitability. Epilepsia 19:567–579, 1978.

8. Burchiel KJ: Effects of electrical and mechanical stimulation on two foci of spontaneous activity which develop in primary afferent neurons after peripheral axotomy. Pain 18:249–265, 1984.

9. Cailliet R: Pain: Mechanisms and Management. Philadelphia, FA Davis, 1993, p 36.

10. Carpenter MB: Core Text of Neuroanatomy. 4th ed. Baltimore, Williams & Wilkins, 1991, p 106.

11. Chester J: Whiplash, postural control, and the inner ear. Spine 16:716–720, 1991.

12. Elvey R: Brachial plexus tension tests and the pathoanatomical origin of arm pain. Proceedings, Aspects of Manipulative Therapy, Lincoln Institute of Health Sciences, Melbourne, 1979, pp 105–110.

13. Gertzbein SD, Tile M, Gross A, et al: Autoimmunity in degenerative disc disease of the lumbar spine. Orthop Clin North Am 6:67–73, 1975.

14. Goldberg ME, Eggers HM, Gouras P: The ocular motor system. In Kandel ER, Schwartz JH, Jessell TM (eds): Principles of Neural Science. 3rd ed. E Norwalk, CT, Appleton & Lange, 1991, p 661.

15. Hagberg C: Electromyography and bite force studies of muscular function and dysfunction in masticatory muscles. Swed Dent J Suppl 37:1–64, 1986.

16. Hassler R, Walker AE: Trigeminal Neuralgia. Pathogenesis and Pathophysiology. Stuttgart, Georg Thiem, 1970.

17. Kandel ER, Schwartz JH, Jessell TM (eds): Principles of Neural Science. 3rd ed. E Norwalk, CT, Appleton & Lange, 1991.

18. Keele CA, Armstrong D: Substances Producing Pain and Itch. London, Edward Arnold Ltd, 1964.

19. Korr IM: Sustained sympathicotonia as a factor in disease. In The Collected Papers of Irvin M. Korr. American Academy of Osteopathy, 1979.

20. Krag MH: Biomechanics of the spine. In Frymoyer J (ed): The Adult Spine. New York, Raven Press, 1991, pp 929–967.

21. La Rocca H: Cervical sprain syndrome. In Frymoyer J (ed): The Adult Spine. New York, Raven Press, 1991, pp 1051–1063.

22. McAfee PC, Regan JJ, Bohlman HH: Cervical cord compression from ossification of the posterior longitudinal ligament in non-Orientals. J Bone Joint Surg [Br] 69:569–575, 1987.

23. Nachemson A: Intradiscal measurements of pH in patients with lumbar rhizopathies. Acta Orthop Scand 40:23–42, 1969.

24. Macnab I: The mechanism of spondylogenic pain. In Hirsch C, Zotterman Y (eds): Cervical Pain. New York, Pergamon Press, 1972, pp 89–95.

25. Parke WW, Watanabe R: The intrinsic vasculature of the lumbosacral nerve roots. Spine 10:508–515, 1985.

26. Payan DG, McGillis JP, Goetzl EJ: Neuroimmunology. Adv Immunol 39:299–323, 1986.

27. Rauschning W: Anatomy and pathology of the cervical spine. In Frymoyer J (ed): The Adult Spine. New York, Raven Press, 1991.

28. Reid JD: Effects of flexion-extension movements of the head and spine upon the spinal cord and nerve roots. J Neurol Neurosurg Psychiatry 23:214, 1960.

29. Rydevik BL: Etiology of sciatica. In Weinstein JN, Wiesel SW (eds): The Lumbar Spine. Philadelphia, WB Saunders, 1990, p 132.

30. Shaw RR: Pancoast's tumor. Ann Thorac Surg 37:343–345, 1984.

31. Sunderland S: Traumatized nerves, roots and ganglia: Musculoskeletal factors and neuropathological consequences. In Korr IM (ed): Neurobiologic Mechanisms of Manipulative Therapy. New York, Plenum Press, 1978, pp 137–166.

32. Weinstein JN: Mechanism of spinal pain: The dorsal root ganglion and its role as a mediator of low back pain. Spine 11:999–1001, 1986.

33. Weinstein JN, Pope M, Schmidt R, et al: Neuropharmacological effects of vibration: An animal model. Spine 13:521–525, 1988.

34. White AA, Panjabi MM: Clinical Biomechanics of the Spine. 2nd ed. Philadelphia, JB Lippincott, 1990.

35. Xiuqing C, Bo Sun, Shizhen Z: Nerves accompanying the vertebral artery and their clinical relevance. Spine 13:1360–1364, 1988.

CHAPTER 3

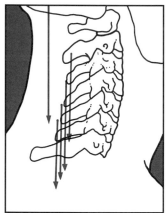

MUSCULATURE OF THE CERVICAL SPINE

Although a significant volume of research has been carried out in the study of ligamentous contributions to cervical spine stability, few investigations have focused on the muscles of this region. A comprehensive study of the function of muscles in the cervical spine includes not only a review of the intricate layering of the various muscles and fascial elements but also an analysis of the contribution of the receptor system within these muscles and an understanding of the coordinated activity between the cervical spine and the respiratory, facial, and oral muscles that are linked by different central nervous system loci in the brain stem and the cervical spinal cord.

One of the objectives of this chapter is to provide the clinician with a three-dimensional orientation to the muscles and fascia of this region and an understanding of their contribution to the dynamic stabilization and mobility demands of the spine. The individual muscles and fascial components of the cervical spine are presented in approximately the same order as they would appear during a dissection of the cervical spine, with the posterior muscles described first, followed by the lateral muscles and, finally, the anterior muscles. This type of organizational scheme provides the clinician with a better understanding of the different layers of muscle encountered with palpa-

tion as well as the relations individual muscles have with surrounding structures.

After a description of the functional anatomy of the muscles and fascia, the important contributions of key muscle receptors—the muscle spindle and tendon organ—are described to illustrate the array of proprioceptive and kinesthetic information available to the central nervous system by way of cervical muscle activity. This is especially pertinent to discussions of the cervical spine musculature because spindles are particularly dense in muscles that interconnect the cervical vertebrae.[7] As discussed below, several of the theories surrounding treatment of the cervical spine are based on attempts to influence the proprioceptive receptors located in cervical spine muscles. Perhaps one of the reasons these treatment strategies are so effective is because the clinician has intuitively recognized that contractile states of the cervical spine muscles can be readily influenced by using various manual techniques. Such techniques are important because they ultimately affect cervical spine motion. The ease with which these techniques can be successfully performed is perhaps due to the fact that the cervical spine muscles feature an extraordinarily dense array of muscle spindles.

In addition to the importance of proprioceptors, the linkage between the cervical spine musculature and the sensory receptors of the head deserves attention. Because of the plethora of reflex connections between the sensory organs of the head and the motor neuron pools related to the cervical spine, the musculature of the neck is required to serve many unique and highly coordinated functions. The patient with cervical spine pain often feels further compromised because he or she cannot move the neck at the desired speed or through the necessary range to optimally position the sense organs such as the eyes and ears.

Until recently, the musculature of the cervical spine was not as well understood as the musculature of the extremities. As a result, treatment techniques for the soft tissues of the neck tended to be more passive than activity-oriented. Although such an approach may be indicated in the very early phases of cervical spine soft tissue injury, it is now recognized that an active approach toward rehabilitation is associated with more positive long-term outcomes. The treatment approach should be as activity-oriented as possible in the later phases of the rehabilitation program to begin to introduce controlled stresses into the soft tissues and to facilitate functional activities. Consequently, the clinician is best served by having a three-dimensional appreciation of the various layers of cervical spine muscles and an understanding of the roles they might play in mobility and stability functions.

NEUROMUSCULAR TREATMENT TECHNIQUES

Before detailing the muscles of the cervical spine, it is perhaps useful to summarize the intent and application technique for three of the most common neuromuscular treatment techniques for the cervical spine. The clinician may use the information that follows to refine and augment the repertoire of manual techniques designed to influence the neuromuscular apparatus of the cervical spine. Such techniques emphasize the direction of muscle fibers, muscle attachments, and relations between the various muscle layers of the cervical spine as well as the influence of the muscle receptor system.

Neuromuscular treatment techniques that use

Table 3–1. Methods of Enhancing Motion in Cervical Spine Disorders Using Muscle Action
Contraction of agonistic muscles
Isometric contraction of antagonists
Reciprocal inhibition of antagonists

the contraction of the cervical spine muscles can be placed within the following three categories (Table 3–1):

1. Contraction of the agonist muscles to actively improve range (active contraction of agonists)

2. Stretching techniques to increase motion of the cervical spine after isometric contraction of antagonistic muscles (isometric contraction of antagonists)

3. Stretching techniques to increase motion after reciprocal inhibition of the antagonistic muscles by means of isometric contraction of the agonist muscles (isometric contraction of agonists)

Optimally, each of these techniques is used for a different purpose and at a different stage of tissue healing. The difference between the techniques also results in different stresses to the muscles themselves.

Active Contraction of Agonists

In the first technique, the clinician has assessed the cervical spine and determined the direction in which a limitation of motion is seen and whether familiar pain is reproduced. Such an assessment includes both active and passive tests (see Chapter 5). This treatment technique is designed to use contraction of those muscles that are considered agonists of the desired motion. The clinician moves the cervical spine to the point of the range-of-motion limitation (also referred to clinically as the barrier), and the patient then attempts to actively move beyond the range-of-motion limitation using active concentric muscle contraction. The clinician may position the head and neck at the limitation of motion and then guide the patient through the process of initiating appropriate muscle contraction to move through and beyond the barrier. This is essentially a self-mobilization technique by the patient.

Because it may be difficult for the patient to begin these new movements, the clinician must assist the patient with the desired muscle contraction and movement pattern. A clinician who has a detailed understanding of the anatomy can often place the head and cervical spine in varied positions to lessen tensile or compressive forces over selected regions while facilitating the desired active muscle contraction to increase range of motion and neuromuscular coordination. Understanding the directions of the muscles, their lines of force, and their relative depth in the cervical spine allows for tactile stimuli to be used effectively to help guide the desired movements.

Isometric Contraction of Antagonists

In the second technique, the impressions gained from the assessment of the head and neck suggest that the motion of the cervical spine is limited because of adaptive shortening of the muscle and connective tissues or that an increased resting tension of the muscle restricts the motion. The clinician analyzes the forces that reproduce familiar pain and makes a determination whether motion should be increased, either by stretching the shortened tissues or by altering the resting state of tension of the cervical spine musculature causing the motion limitation. Careful attention must be given to analyzing this aspect of the assessment because an increase in muscle tension may be an appropriate response of neuromuscular guarding designed to protect injured tissues.

If a decision is made to attempt to increase motion, the cervical spine motion is taken to the barrier, and the technique requires that an isometric contraction of the involved cervical spine musculature be initiated. After the relaxation phase, a passive stretching force to move past the barrier is imparted by the clinician. In this case, the isometric contraction would be in a direction *away* from the direction of motion limitation followed by a stretching maneuver *into* the motion barrier. It is important to realize, however, that this technique places a tensile force through the musculature on two counts: the isometric contraction of the muscle and the subsequent stretch. Such a technique would be contraindicated in the early phases of soft tissue healing after an acceleration injury to the neck, for example. Once again, the ability to analyze the direction of the muscles of the cervical spine optimizes the chance for a successful treatment outcome in both the isometric contraction and the stretching phases of the technique.

Isometric Contraction of Agonists

In the third treatment technique, the principle of reciprocal inhibition is used to increase cervical spine motion. During the assessment, the clinician determines the direction of motion limitation, and how this limitation contributes to the painful syndrome. The cervical spine is taken to the motion barrier, and an isometric contraction of the musculature is initiated by the patient *in the direction of* the motion limitation. The resistance to such a motion must be applied by the clinician in a specific direction and intensity and with great care. Contraction of the musculature in this manner affords reflex relaxation of the antagonistic muscle groups, which subsequently are stretched by the clinician. A tensile force is placed on the involved cervical spine musculature only during the stretching phase of the treatment, which is an important difference between this technique and the second technique. Again, a detailed understanding of the direction, attachments, and lines of force of the musculature optimizes the chance for a successful treatment outcome.

These three treatment approaches are just a few of the variations possible in working with the muscles of the cervical spine. Such techniques also impart mechanical stresses to connective tissues related to the muscles, cervical joints, and intervertebral discs. For example, because many of the muscles of the cervical spine cross several segments, their contraction results in compressive forces to the apophyseal joints and between the vertebral bodies and intervertebral discs (Fig. 3–1). Likewise, the direction of muscle fibers can also result in anterior or posterior shear forces between the apophyseal joint surfaces and the vertebral body–intervertebral disc interface (Fig. 3–2).

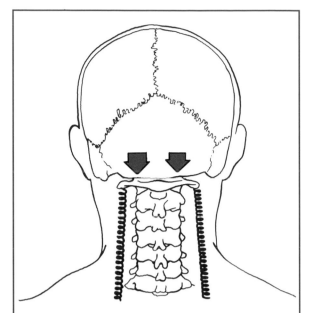

Figure 3–1. The action of the musculature results in compression to the vertebral segments as well as movement.

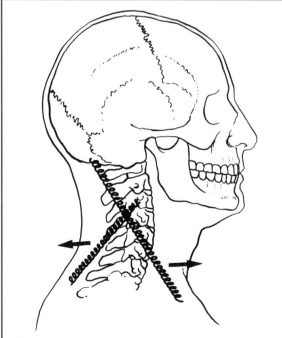

Figure 3–2. Contraction of the musculature results in anterior or posterior shear forces on the cervical spine.

IMPORTANCE OF COORDINATED, PAIN-FREE MOVEMENT OF THE CERVICAL SPINE

One of the differences between the head–cervical–upper thoracic spine complex and the lower thoracic–lumbar–pelvic complex is in the local demands of stability and mobility. In the low back region, a greater emphasis often is placed on muscle training to enhance stability of this region and to condition the muscular system to help attenuate ground and trunk forces that converge into the low back.

The demands on the neuromuscular apparatus in the neck are different, however, because of the need to continually reposition the sense organs. Mobility of the neck is important because head and neck postures often are rapidly assumed to optimize the position of sense organs such as the eyes and ears. For example, in attempting to track an object with the eyes, it is essential that there be a concurrent, coordinated contraction of the cervical spine musculature to allow the eyes to follow the object. Likewise, when people are subjected to a sound, they often reflexively position the head and neck to improve the chances of the sound waves reaching the auditory apparatus. In addition, they may attempt to direct the eyes toward the source of the sound by means of rapid head and neck positioning.

These motions of the cervical spine are subtle, but they are smooth and occur rapidly and, in most instances, without conscious effort. The speed with which such postural adaptations occur in response to visual and auditory stimuli is due to reflex connections between the sensory and auditory apparati and the motor neuron pools in the cervical spinal cord and brain stem.

Clinically, it is the inability to rapidly position the head and neck or to place the head and neck in pain-free positions that is a major complaint. A rapid, reflexive movement of the head and neck can dramatically increase pain if tissues are injured. A simple activity such as looking over one's shoulder when backing a car out of a driveway or holding the head and neck in a fixed position and initiating small, subtle neck motions while reading becomes a frustrating task for the patient. For this reason, mobility and coordination deficits—especially those that exacerbate the painful syndrome—assume great importance in cervical spine disorders and help to illustrate why the clinician must have detailed knowledge of the musculature of the cervical spine.

The coordination between the cervical spine muscles and the oral-facial muscles should also be emphasized. For the muscles of the mandible to actively and rhythmically open and close the mouth, the occiput must be stabilized, with subtle changes in position and fixation continuously occurring. In addition, the position of the cervical spine and occiput helps to determine how the maxillary and mandibular teeth make contact with each other. Mobility, coordination, and the ability to rapidly assume and maintain various head and neck postures are thus of primary importance in relation to the cervical spine.

Muscles related to the scapula should be viewed in the context of their primary functions. Strength, endurance, and postural stability are important qualities of the musculature related to the scapula because of the influence of scapulothoracic mechanics on postural mechanics of both the shoulder girdle and the head and neck.

This aspect is discussed in further detail in subsequent sections dealing with individual muscles.

FASCIA OF THE CERVICAL SPINE

As in other areas of the musculoskeletal system, the fascial network is intimately related to the muscles of the cervical spine. Fascia plays an important role in directing the force of muscle contraction through the weight-bearing tissues such as the articular cartilage of the apophyseal joints and vertebral body–intervertebral disc interface. Besides serving as aponeurotic attachments for the muscles, the fascia encases muscles and organizes the muscles into different fascial planes.

The fascia of the cervical spine appears highly complex at first but is organized along an understandable framework. Fascial planes are used extensively to guide surgical approaches to the neck, and an awareness of their relations to surrounding structures is important for the clinician to understand the unique compartments related to the cervical spine.

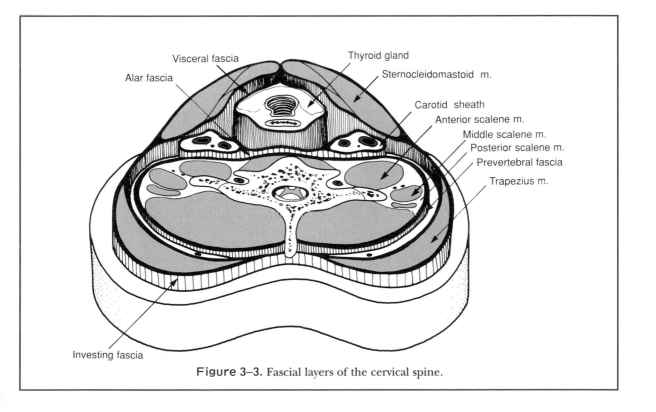

Figure 3–3. Fascial layers of the cervical spine.

Immediately beneath the skin on the anterior aspect of the neck are the superficial fascia and fat, in which are housed the two platysma muscles. Just deep to this superficial fascia is the investing fascia, sometimes referred to as the superficial layer of deep cervical fascia (Fig. 3–3). This investing layer should not be confused with the superficial fascia that houses the platysma but rather should be recognized as an extensive fascial investment that surrounds the neck.

The remaining layers of cervical fascia are as follows (see Fig. 3–3):

1. Fascia that surrounds the short *strap muscles* in the anterior neck (those muscles related to the hyoid bone and thyroid cartilage)

2. *Visceral fascia,* which surrounds the larynx, trachea, esophagus, and thyroid

3. *Alar fascia,* which is immediately behind the esophagus and spreads laterally to surround structures within the carotid sheath

4. *Prevertebral fascia,* which surrounds the vertebral bodies and muscles anteriorly and continues laterally and posteriorly to cover the paraspinal cervical muscles. This layer of fascia is continuous with the thoracolumbar fascia of the low back.

Investing Fascia

The investing fascia is a thick, tough layer of connective tissue, the extent of which is not often appreciated during palpation of the cervical spine. It is attached to the large ligamentum nuchae and all the cervical spinous processes, courses laterally to invest the trapezius muscle, and continues anteriorly to also invest the sternocleidomastoid muscle. The investing fascia from both sides meets anteriorly at the midline. Figure 3–3 shows how this fascia simultaneously encircles the cervical spine tissues and envelopes both the trapezius and the sternocleidomastoid muscle, hence the term *investing*. While remaining superficial to the posterior vertebral muscles, it encases these two superficial muscles.

Inferiorly, the investing fascia is attached to the spine of the scapula, acromion process, clavicle, and manubrium. Superiorly, it blends with the periosteum over the external occipital protuberance, superior nuchal line, and mastoid process of the temporal bone. Thus, this fascial complex is attached superiorly to the occiput and inferiorly to the bones related to the shoulder girdle. With such an arrangement, one can begin to appreciate the fact that the investing fascia forms a connective tissue encasement for the complete cervical spine.

POSTERIOR MUSCLES OF THE CERVICAL SPINE

Trapezius Muscle

Separating the posterior layer of the investing fascia from the underlying trapezius muscle is difficult because the deep surface of the investing fascia serves as an attachment for much of the trapezius muscle tissue (Fig. 3–4). The intimate relation between the trapezius muscle and the investing fascia often is not appreciated. Note how the contraction and subsequent broadening of the trapezius muscle have the potential to place an expansion type of force on the investing fascia because the broadening muscle is contained within this envelope. In addition, contraction of the trapezius muscle places tensile forces through the investing layer of fascia by way of the attachments to the inner walls of this fascia.

The investing fascia in the upper cervical spine typically is thicker than that over the region of the middle trapezius. When the fascia is carefully removed from its attachment at the nuchal line toward the mastoid process, the sternocleidomastoid insertion can be seen covering the insertion of the splenius capitis muscle. This insertional region related to the mastoid process is discussed in a later section because it serves as a major point of attachment for several muscles and the investing fascia. It also is subject to significant tensile forces and often is an area of palpable tenderness and discomfort in patients with head and neck pain. The region is mentioned at this point to provide the reader with an understanding of muscular relations between the trapezius and surrounding muscles at the occiput.

It is important to recognize the prominent tendinous region of the trapezius over the lower cervical and upper thoracic spinous processes (Fig. 3–5). Although the trapezius muscle often is pictured as consisting completely of muscle tissue from the occiput to the lower thoracic spine, this

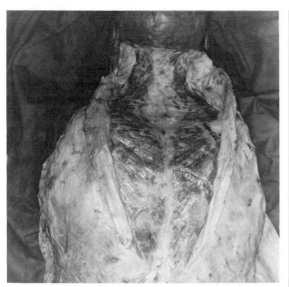
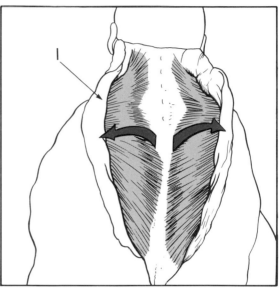

Figure 3–4. Investing layer of fascia (I). This fascial layer must be removed before the superficial muscles are seen.

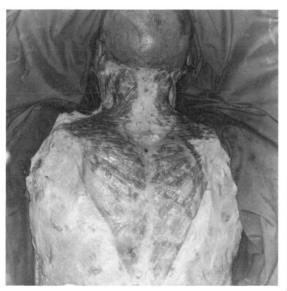
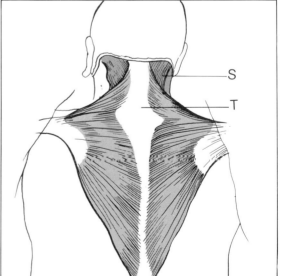

Figure 3–5. Tendinous attachment of the trapezius at the cervicothoracic junction. S, splenius capitis muscle; T, tendinous attachment of the trapezius muscle at the region of the cervicothoracic junction.

in fact seldom is the case. The muscle has a broad connective tissue, nonmuscular component over the region of the cervicothoracic junction.

The trapezius muscle has a broad region of attachment to the occiput, ligamentum nuchae, and thoracic spinous processes and laterally to the spine of the scapula, acromion, and lateral third of the clavicle. In many cases, the muscle does not reach the occiput but attaches to it indirectly by way of its attachment to the ligamentum nuchae. The central aspect of the trapezius muscle over the region of the lower cervical and upper thoracic spinous, which consists of connective tissue rather than muscle tissue, is shown in Figure 3–5.

Actions of the trapezius are discussed after a review of the sternocleidomastoid muscle, but it is important to recognize that the trapezius is primarily a muscle of the shoulder girdle and essentially connects the shoulder girdle to the vertebral column. If the upper limb is strongly fixated, the trapezius can extend the head on the cervical spine.

Conversely, for the trapezius muscle to elevate the scapula, the occiput and cervical spine must be fixated to assure the proper transference of force to the scapula. Fixation of the occiput in this case would be due to action of two anteriorly placed muscles, the longus capitis and longus colli. These muscles help to fixate the head and neck and prevent an extension motion. With the head and neck dynamically fixated in such a manner, the trapezius muscle can use the stabilized occiput as an anchor from which to elevate the scapula (Fig. 3–6). This synergy between the longus colli and capitis and the trapezius muscles helps to explain why the acceleration injury of the neck, which results in an uncontrolled extension force with excessive tensile stress to the anterior neck musculature, results in a marked inability of patients to elevate their shoulders in a pain-free manner. In these syndromes, the injured longus colli and capitis cannot fixate the head and neck, and thus the trapezius cannot pull from a stabilized occiput.

The intricate neural mechanisms that control head, neck, and scapular motions can also be appreciated when the levator scapulae and upper trapezius muscle functions are compared. Both muscles have the potential to elevate the shoulder girdle, and thus they act as synergists for this activity. In contrast, complete abduction of the

shoulder requires an upward rotation movement of the scapula. When the scapula is rotated upward, the upper trapezius is actively shortened and a lengthening contraction occurs with the levator scapulae muscle. Therefore, with abduction of the shoulder, the same two muscles now work as antagonists.

Travell and Simons consider the trapezius muscle to be the cervical spine muscle most often beset by trigger points, with such trigger points often being a source of irritation leading to temporal headache.[17] They further suggest that pain

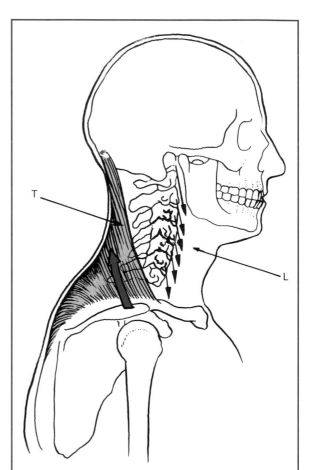

Figure 3–6. Sagittal view of the cervical spine showing the synergistic relation between the trapezius and the longus capitis and colli. The longus capitis must prevent the occiput from extending for the trapezius to use this fixed origin from which to elevate the shoulder girdle. L, Force vectors of the longus colli and capitis muscles; T, trapezius.

on motion caused by upper trapezius trigger points occurs when the head and neck are fully rotated to the opposite side of pain because this contracts the muscle into a fully shortened position.

Sternocleidomastoid Muscle

The sternocleidomastoid muscle is intimately related to the investing fascia (Fig. 3–7). This is an important muscle clinically because it usually is one of the anterior soft tissue structures injured during an acceleration injury. McNab has identified tears in the sternocleidomastoid muscle as the most common lesion that occurs during an acceleration injury when the impact is from behind, followed by damage to the longus colli muscle and anterior longitudinal ligaments and separation of the intervertebral discs from the vertebral bodies.[10]

Ashton-Miller and colleagues demonstrated experimentally that referred pain patterns from the sternocleidomastoid muscle, occurring as a result of a hypertonic saline solution injection to the muscle, primarily ascended along the muscle and became diffuse in the temporomandibular area.[1]

Muscle pain from the sternocleidomastoid also resulted in increased motor output in both the relaxed and the active state of the muscle and altered the motor output to the synergists and antagonists of the sternocleidomastoid. It has also been suggested that trigger points in the sternocleidomastoid muscle have the potential to initiate autonomic eye responses such as lacrimation, ptosis, and visual disturbances as well as induce postural and spatial disturbances such as dizziness and vertigo.[17]

The sternocleidomastoid and trapezius muscles have identical relations to the investing fascia as well as attachments to bones related to the shoulder girdle: the trapezius to the scapula and clavicle and the sternocleidomastoid to the clavicle and manubrium of the sternum.

In addition, both muscles have a similar innervation pattern in that they are supplied by cranial nerve XI, the spinal accessory nerve. The portion of the motor nerve responsible for innervation of the trapezius and sternocleidomastoid actually arises from ventral roots of the cervical spinal cord located within the spinal canal. These nerve fibers ascend within the canal through the foramen magnum to briefly enter the cranial cavity

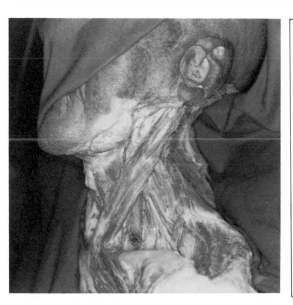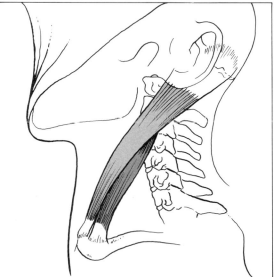

Figure 3–7. Muscle belly and attachments of the sternocleidomastoid muscle.

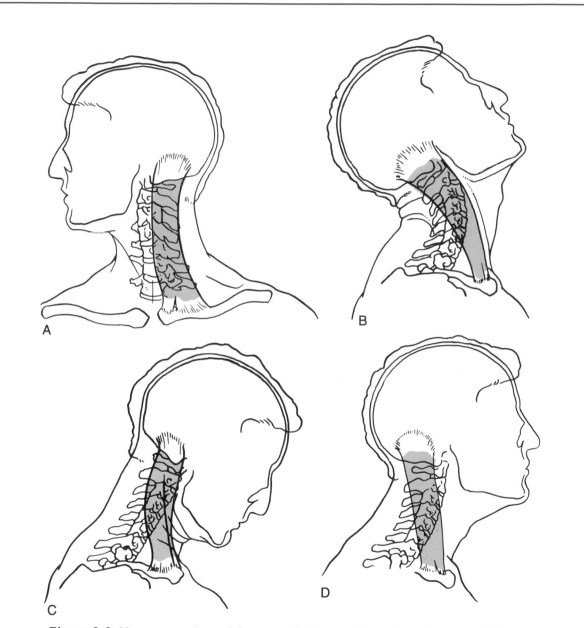

Figure 3–8. Numerous actions of the sternocleidomastoid muscle. *A,* Rotation. *B,* Upper part of the sternocleidomastoid causing extension of the upper spine. *C,* Lower part of the sternocleidomastoid causing flexion of the lower cervical spine. *D,* Bilateral contraction resulting in forward-head translation as well as anterior shear. The upper portion of the sternocleidomastoid muscle can also exert an extension moment on the occiput-atlas articulation.

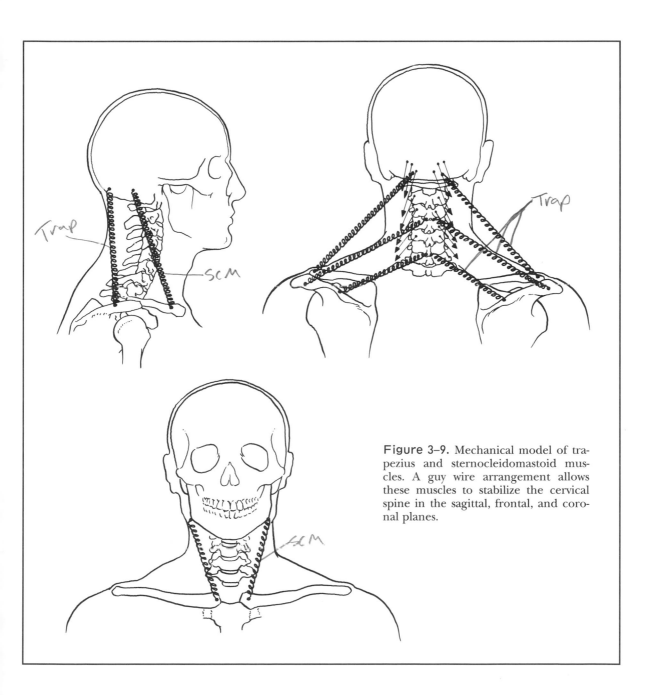

Figure 3–9. Mechanical model of trapezius and sternocleidomastoid muscles. A guy wire arrangement allows these muscles to stabilize the cervical spine in the sagittal, frontal, and coronal planes.

and then exit the skull through the jugular foramen to supply the sternocleidomastoid and trapezius muscles.

The sternocleidomastoid muscle passes obliquely across the side of the neck. It is thicker in the central region and then thins and broadens at its superior attachment to the mastoid process and inferior attachment to the sternum and clavicle. Because it is a superficial structure and easily visualized through the skin, it can serve the clinician as an important indicator of a forward-head posture. The greater the verticality of the sternocleidomastoid muscle when the neck is viewed in the sagittal plane, the greater the likelihood that a forward-head posture is present.

The sternocleidomastoid muscle has many individualized functions (Fig. 3–8). Its oblique course in passing from sternal origin to mastoid insertion allows it to cause rotation at most of the cervical segments. Because the upper portion of the muscle is posterior to the center of rotation for flexion and extension of the cervical spine and the inferior portion of the muscle is anterior to this center of rotation, the sternocleidomastoid has the potential to extend the upper cervical segments, especially the occiput on the atlas, and flex the lower cervical segments.

Perhaps more important, the lower aspects of the sternocleidomastoid muscles are oriented to resist forceful extension or backward movement of the cervical spine, which is one of the reasons they become injured with an acceleration injury of the neck that forcefully extends the cervical spine. The two sternocleidomastoid muscles form important anterior and lateral guys for the head and neck, and their contraction causes a relative forward translation of the cervical spine with an anterior shear force imparted between the joint surfaces.

The trapezius and sternocleidomastoid muscles have attachments located a significant distance from the center of rotation for the cervical spine. Therefore, they have longer lever arms than most of the other cervical muscles. This allows these muscles to serve as efficient guy wires in the sagittal, frontal, and coronal planes (Fig. 3–9). Although they do not form a complete muscular envelope around the cervical spine like the investing layer of cervical fascia, the trapezius and sternocleidomastoid muscles nearly encircle the neck, usually being separated only by the invest-

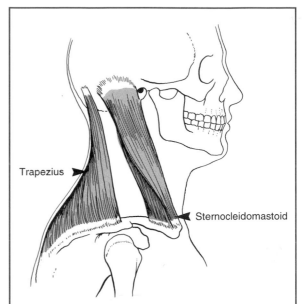

Figure 3–10. The sternocleidomastoid and trapezius muscles almost encircle the neck. A muscle-fascia collar is formed by the investing fascia, trapezius muscles, and sternocleidomastoid muscles.

ing fascia, which covers the posterior triangle of the neck (Fig. 3–10). When viewed together in such a manner, these two similarly innervated muscles offer dynamic synergistic support to the underlying soft tissues and visceral structures in the neck.

Rhomboid Major and Minor and Levator Scapulae Muscles

When the trapezius muscle is reflected from its attachments to the cervical and thoracic spinous processes, the rhomboid major muscle can be seen attaching to the medial border of the scapula; the rhomboid minor muscle, to the root of the spine of the scapula; and the levator scapulae muscle, to the superior angle of the scapula (Fig. 3–11). In contrast to the muscular attachments to the scapula, the attachment of the rhomboid muscles to the spinous processes typically is tendinous (Fig. 3–12).

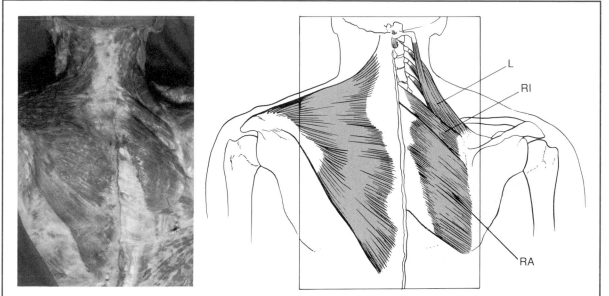

Figure 3–11. Frontal plane, posterior view of the rhomboid major and minor and the levator scapulae. L, levator scapulae muscle; RA, rhomboid major muscle; RI, rhomboid minor muscle.

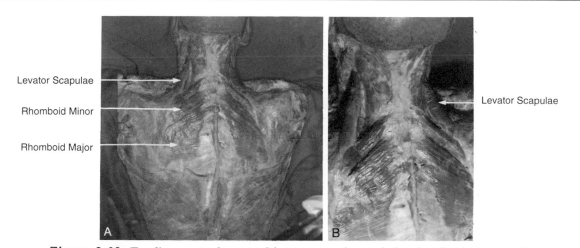

Figure 3–12. Tendinous attachment of levator scapulae and the rhomboid major and minor muscles.

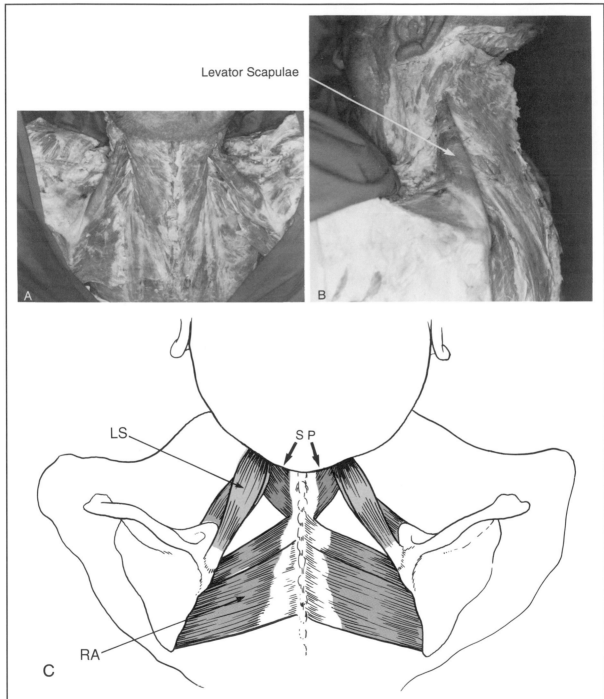

Figure 3–13. *A–C,* View of the levator scapulae showing the suspensory capacity of this large muscle of the cervical spine. LS, levator scapulae muscle; RA, rhomboid major muscle; SP, spenius capitis.

The frontal plane view of the levator scapulae, as shown in Figure 3–11, does not adequately illustrate the multiple functions of this muscle. The levator scapulae muscle courses superiorly, medially, and anteriorly to reach the cervical transverse processes. The significant anterior inclination is not often appreciated in a frontal plane view, but this orientation allows the muscle to play an important role in cervical spine mechanics. The levator scapulae muscle commonly is large and presents a much more significant cross section than the rhomboid muscles. Figure 3–13 shows how the cervical spine is suspended from the scapula through the muscular strut of the large levator scapulae.

The levator scapulae muscle usually is described as a scapula elevator and lateral flexor of the neck because of its attachments to the cervical transverse processes. It is also optimally aligned to direct a posterior shear force to the vertebrae of the cervical spine. In this regard, it is reasonable to compare the fiber direction, attachments, and function of the levator scapulae to those of the deep erector spinae (also referred to as the lumbar portion of the erector spinae) of the low back. The deep erector spinae muscles arise from the ilium just lateral to the posterior superior iliac spine and course anteriorly, medially, and superiorly to attach to the lumbar transverse processes. They help to actively counter anterior shear that occurs as a result of gravitational force on the lumbar lordosis.[12] In a patient with suspected lumbar spinal instability, the deep erector spinae muscles are required to maintain a continuous state of contraction to counter the gravitational force to the lumbar lordosis, which results in anterior shear of the lumbar vertebrae. Thus tenderness to palpation often can be elicited over the region just lateral to the posterior superior iliac spine and the adjacent ilium, which serves as the point of attachment for the deep erector spinae muscles.

In the same manner, the levator scapulae muscle takes origin from the superomedial border of the scapula and courses anteriorly, medially, and superiorly to attach to the cervical transverse processes. The cervical spine is also subject to the anterior shear force resulting from the pull of gravity caused by the cervical lordosis, and the levator scapulae is oriented to help provide a dynamic restraint to this force. A forward-head posture accentuates the anterior shear force at the cervical spine, and this posture obliges the levator scapulae to maintain a continuous contractile state to dynamically minimize this force.

The superomedial border of the scapula often is tender to palpation in patients with neck pain (just as the region of the posterior superior iliac spine is tender to palpation in a patient with back pain). The mechanics of injury and posture combined with the results of the assessment help to determine whether excessive or prolonged contraction of the levator scapulae to stabilize the cervical spine is contributing to the painful syndrome.

Palpation of the levator scapulae muscle can be facilitated by rotating the head and neck toward the opposite side of the muscle being examined. Because of the attachments of the levator scapulae (transverse processes) and the trapezius (spinous processes), such a rotational maneuver increases tension on the levator scapulae but decreases tension on the trapezius. For example, if the left levator scapulae is being examined, rotation of the neck to the right causes the left transverse process to move forward, which increases tension on the left levator scapulae muscle. The same rotation results in movement of the spinous process toward the left, which decreases tension of the left trapezius. The tautness palpated therefore probably reflects the contractile state of the muscular tissue of the levator scapulae under the overlying relaxed trapezius.

When increased tension is palpated, caution should be used against immediately concluding that the muscle needs to be stretched. Depending on the mechanics of injury, the stage of healing, and the ability of the injured tissue to attenuate the various forces that reach the region, muscle guarding may in fact be an appropriate neuromuscular response to the injury. Rather than immediately stretching the muscle, it may be more logical to consider ways to minimize the anterior shear force occurring over the cervical spine, thus helping to decrease the demands on the levator scapulae muscle.

The scapula provides a base of attachment for the levator scapulae. Because the scapula is not fixed like the pelvis, the position of the scapula is maintained in part by the control of muscles such as the trapezius and the rhomboid major and minor. These three muscles have a scapular retrac-

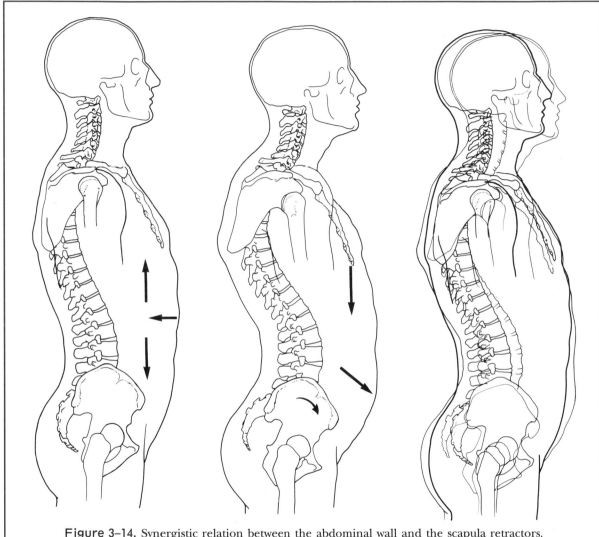

Figure 3–14. Synergistic relation between the abdominal wall and the scapula retractors. Weakness of the abdominal wall results in the inferior collapse of the chest. This change in abdomen-chest relationship places the scapulae in a more protracted position with a resultant lengthening of the scapular retractors.

tion function, and the upper and lower trapezius have a scapular elevation and depression function, respectively. Scapular fixation also results from the action of the serratus anterior muscle.

A rounded-shoulder posture commonly is attributed to the lengthening or weakness of the scapular retractors. Attention should also be given, however, to the role the abdominal wall muscles play as they work synergistically with the scapula retractors, diaphragm, and pelvic floor muscles to align the abdomen and thorax as well as to the relation of the scapula to the thorax (Fig. 3–14). Weakness of the abdominal muscles results in the sternum and chest being carried more caudally, which accentuates the rounded-shoulder posture. Scapular retractor strengthening, scapulothoracic postural positioning, and abdominal wall training provide a more complete treatment approach for the forward-head, rounded-shoulder posture.

Another important action of the rhomboid major and minor muscles is deceleration of the scapula during protraction movements of the scapula, such as those motions that occur during throwing. In this instance, the thoracic spine must be stabilized so that the rhomboid muscles can use the spinous process attachments as anchors for the eccentric contraction necessary to control scapular movement. Such activity illustrates the synergistic relation between the muscles of the thoracic spine and the scapula decelerators, such as the rhomboids.

Prevertebral Fascia and the Splenius Muscles

With the investing fascia and trapezius muscle removed from the posterior aspect of the neck, the next layer of fascia encountered is the prevertebral fascia (see Fig. 3–3). As does the investing fascia, the prevertebral fascia encircles the neck, but it is related to the deeper muscles and is continuous with the thoracolumbar fascia of the low back. The prevertebral fascia covers the splenius and semispinalis muscle groups posteriorly and attaches to the occiput with these mus-cles. It then courses laterally to cover the scalene muscles and anteriorly to cover the longus colli and capitis muscles (see Fig. 3–3).

The splenius capitis and splenius cervicis are large flat muscles that course from the cervical and thoracic spinous process and ligamentum nuchae and extend upward and lateral to attach to the superior nuchal line and mastoid process (capitis portion) and the posterior tubercles of the cervical transverse processes (cervicis portion) (Fig. 3–15). The mastoid process attachment of the splenius capitis deserves special mention. This site serves as an important attachment for several large muscles. From superficial to deep, they are the sternocleidomastoid, splenius capitis, and longissimus capitis muscles. The sternocleidomastoid has already been described, and the longissimus group is discussed below. Note at this time, however, the significant force that can be exerted to the mastoid process because of these three muscle attachments.

The splenius capitis has an excellent lever arm for cervical extension because of its attachment to the occiput, and the lateral course of its muscle fibers from the spinous processes toward the occiput make it well suited to rotation of the

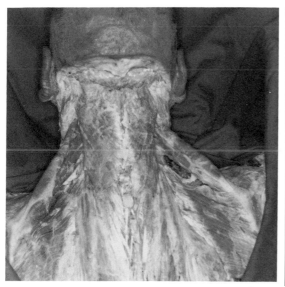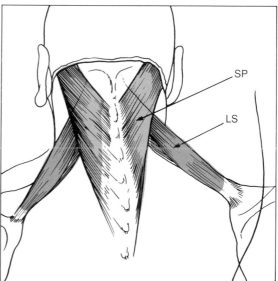

Figure 3–15. Splenius capitis muscle. LS, levator scapulae muscle; SP, splenius capitis muscle.

cervical spine. This rotary function is due to its attachments to the posterior tubercle of the cervical transverse processes (cervicis portion) and mastoid process (capitis portion), which affords the muscle a mechanically advantageous lever arm. Rotation occurs to the same side as the contracting muscle. Working bilaterally, the splenius capitis shows strong activity during extension of the head and neck with almost no activity in the upright balanced antigravity posture.[16]

Semispinalis Muscle Group

When the broad, flat splenius capitis muscle is removed from its attachments to the cervical and thoracic spinous processes and reflected laterally, it is seen to cover the underlying semispinalis capitis and longissimus capitis muscles. In this section, the semispinalis muscles are considered.

The semispinalis cervicis and capitis muscles are perhaps the most important extensor muscles of the occiput and cervical spine because their muscle fibers are oriented to generate a line of force that results in nearly pure extension of the cervical spine and the occiput.[11] By virtue of their attachments to the occiput and cervical spinous processes, the semispinalis muscles cause posterior sagittal rotation of the cervical vertebrae— extension of the cervical spine—which in effect is an increase in the cervical lordosis. This is a much different action than just bringing the head and neck in a posterior direction, an action that does not necessarily result in posterior sagittal rotation of the vertebrae or an increase in the cervical lordosis.

The semispinalis cervicis and capitis are relatively massive muscles of the cervical spine with exceptionally broad and thick tendons. The semispinalis cervicis muscles attach to the tips of the cervical spinous processes, especially at the region of the second cervical vertebra; the semispinalis capitis has a strong attachment to the occiput (Fig. 3–16). These attachments place the complete semispinalis group well posterior to the center of rotation of cervical spine motion, providing a long lever arm for cervical spine extension. The semispinalis cervicis and capitis muscles are such important extensors of the cervical spine that it has been recommended that any surgical procedures for the posterior aspect of the cervical spine should minimally disrupt these muscles because removal of the muscles and incorrect re-

alignment may result in loss of normal cervical alignment.[11] They are considered the prime movers for increasing and dynamically maintaining the cervical lordosis.

The semispinalis cervicis muscle arises from the transverse processes of the upper thoracic vertebrae and courses superiorly to attach to the spinous processes of the second through fifth cervical vertebrae, with the attachment to the spinous process of the axis (C2) being the largest portion of the muscle. Such a significant attachment to the spinous process of the axis suggests the important stabilizing effect this muscle has on the second cervical vertebra so that two of the larger suboccipital muscles, the inferior oblique and rectus capitis posterior major muscles, can then act over the atlas-axis and occiput-axis articulations, respectively.

The semispinalis capitis muscle nearly covers the semispinalis cervicis. It arises from the transverse processes of the upper thoracic vertebrae and lower cervical vertebrae and from the articular processes of the lower cervical spine, often by a thick, strong tendon, and then courses directly cranialward to attach to the occiput between the superior and inferior nuchal lines (see Fig. 3–16). In the cervical region, the muscle is covered by the trapezius and splenius capitis muscles and their related fascial coverings.

Because the semispinalis capitis overlies the semispinalis cervicis, the combined morphology of the two muscles attains a more rounded, fusiform shape. Therefore, these muscles may be perceived by the clinician as the rounded muscle bundle immediately lateral to the cervical spinous processes during palpation of the neck because by comparison, the splenius and trapezius muscles are flat. The two semispinalis muscles occupy the region just lateral to the nuchal ligament and spinous processes of the cervical spine, directly over the lamina of the cervical vertebrae. This paraspinal location, combined with their fusiform shape and large cross section, makes them readily accessible for palpation.

Figure 3–16 also shows the manner in which the greater occipital nerve pierces the semispinalis capitis muscle. Travell and Simons suggest that an entrapment syndrome of the greater occipital nerve is caused by hyperirritability of the semispinalis capitis muscles.[17] Pain and numbness or a burning sensation over the scalp and occipital region are typical symptoms of greater occipital

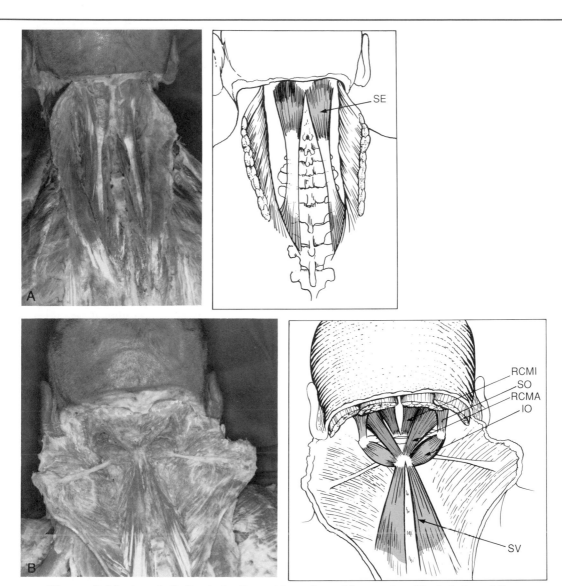

Figure 3–16. *A* and *B,* Semispinalis capitis and cervicis muscles. IO, inferior oblique muscle; RCMA, rectus capitis posterior major muscle; RCMI, rectus capitis posterior minor muscle; SE, semispinalis capitis muscle; SO, superior oblique muscle; SV, semispinalis cervicis muscle.

nerve entrapment. This type of symptomatology (burning or numbness) is different in quality from the referred pain that stems from cervical joint or intervertebral disc pathology.

There is remarkable similarity between the multifidus muscles in the lumbar spine and the semispinalis muscles in the cervical spine in terms of structure and function. Each muscle is described as a transversospinalis muscle in anatomy textbooks, but such a description is not totally adequate because it implies that a rotatory function is their primary role. Instead, the attachment to the spinous processes provides both muscles with an optimal lever arm for extension of the spine or, more specifically, posterior sagittal rotation of the lumbar or cervical vertebrae. Although there is a separate muscular entity known as the multifidus muscles in the cervical spine, they are extremely small in this region and appear closely applied to the sides of the spinous processes. When function is considered as well as the relative size of the muscles, a more logical comparison is between the multifidus muscles in the lumbar spine and the semispinalis muscles in the cervical spine.

The clinician does not often have an appreciation of the impressive cross section of lumbar multifidus and the semispinalis muscles, but when they are seen by way of dissection, their role as major extensors of the lumbar and cervical spine, respectively, is better appreciated (Fig. 3–17). Both muscles have fascicles that overlap and cross either one segment (deeper fascicles) or several segments (superficial fascicles). The layers, much like overlapping tiles of a roof, provide these muscles with their bulk. Figure 3–18 shows the relative cross-sectional area of the attachment of the semispinalis capitis to the skull. This area should be compared with the rather limited cross-sectional area of the trapezius.

When analyzing muscle forces resulting in cervical spine motion, the clinician is best served by considering the semispinalis group with the small underlying multifidus as one complex. This allows a better appreciation of the function of these muscles during cervical extension motions. In addition, these muscles can be considered to work with the longus colli and capitis as sagittal plane guys controlling the extension and flexion motions of the cervical vertebrae or, more precisely, the posterior and anterior sagittal rotations of the cervical vertebrae that increase or decrease the cervical lordosis. An understanding of the relation between these muscles allows a more spe-

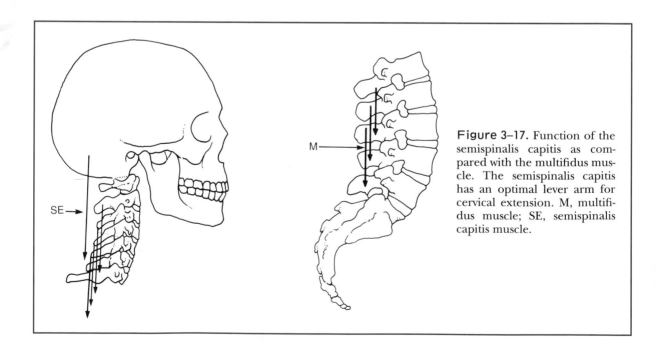

Figure 3–17. Function of the semispinalis capitis as compared with the multifidus muscle. The semispinalis capitis has an optimal lever arm for cervical extension. M, multifidus muscle; SE, semispinalis capitis muscle.

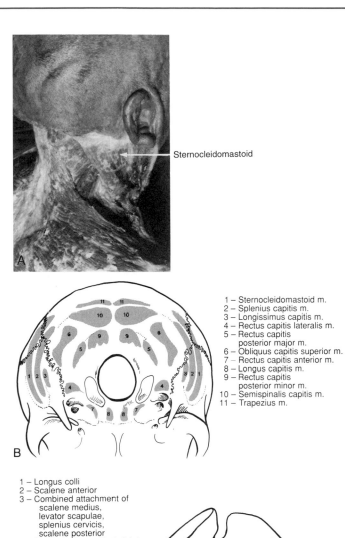

Sternocleidomastoid

1 – Sternocleidomastoid m.
2 – Splenius capitis m.
3 – Longissimus capitis m.
4 – Rectus capitis lateralis m.
5 – Rectus capitis
      posterior major m.
6 – Obliquus capitis superior m.
7 – Rectus capitis anterior m.
8 – Longus capitis m.
9 – Rectus capitis
      posterior minor m.
10 – Semispinalis capitis m.
11 – Trapezius m.

1 – Longus colli
2 – Scalene anterior
3 – Combined attachment of
      scalene medius,
      levator scapulae,
      splenius cervicis,
      scalene posterior
4 – Semispinalis capitis (origin)
5 – Semispinalis cervicis

Figure 3–18. *A,* Cadaver photograph showing the attachment at the mastoid process of the sternocleidomastoid, splenius capitis, and longissimus capitis. *B,* Attachments of muscles to the base of the occiput. *C,* Attachments of muscles to the cervical vertebrae.

cific neuromuscular treatment approach using muscle contraction into or away from the physiological barrier (as described above) to be used.

Longissimus Group

Two muscle groups are uncovered when the broad splenius capitis is reflected: the more medially placed semispinalis group described above and the more laterally placed longissimus muscles. Two portions of the longissimus group are relevant to the cervical region: the longissimus cervicis and the longissimus capitis. The longissimus cervicis courses from the upper thoracic transverse processes to most of the posterior tubercles of the cervical transverse processes. These small tubercles represent the point of attachment for several muscles that appear to blend together: the splenius cervicis, levator scapulae, posterior scalene, and longissimus capitis (see Fig. 3–18). The longissimus capitis muscle courses from the upper thoracic transverse processes and the posterior tubercles of the lower cervical transverse processes to the mastoid process to attach deep to the splenius capitis and sternocleidomastoid muscles.

The attachment of the longissimus capitis muscle to the occiput deserves special mention. The mastoid process is an easily palpated, prominent bony structure. The longissimus capitis, semispinalis capitis, and sternocleidomastoid muscles are attached to this region, and therefore the mastoid process is the focus of significant muscle forces (see Fig. 3–18). Not only should the attachment site be considered an area for potential injury as a result of acceleration, but significant muscle guarding due to a painful syndrome of the neck renders this area vulnerable to pain owing to excessive or prolonged muscle guarding. This is because these three muscles—all with unique and different functions owing to their markedly different lines of muscle force—work to stabilize the neck in all three cardinal planes. The importance of these muscle attachments should be considered when palpation of the mastoid process reveals this region to be painful on examination.

The longissimus muscles are not as large as the semispinalis group and are attached fairly close to the axis of rotation for flexion and extension.

Consequently, they do not have the same mechanical advantage as other muscles that cause extension of the cervical spine. Instead, their laterally placed position aligns them for lateral flexion of the cervical spine and allows the longissimus muscles to serve as lateral guys to help stabilize the head and neck in the frontal plane.

Suboccipital Muscles

When the semispinalis capitis muscle is dissected from its insertion on the occiput and reflected caudally, the suboccipital triangle is exposed (Fig. 3–19). The triangle is formed by the arrangement of the small muscles related to the occiput, atlas, and axis. In the midline are the rectus muscles: rectus capitis posterior minor and rectus capitis posterior major. The rectus capitis posterior major muscle is lateral to and partly covers the minor muscle. It originates from the spine of the axis and ascends to the occiput. The rectus capitis posterior minor starts from the posterior arch of the atlas and ascends to the occiput. These muscles form the most medial aspect of the suboccipital triangle.

The large inferior oblique muscle has a broad origin from the spinous process of the axis and adjacent lamina and travels anteriorly and laterally to attach to the transverse process of the atlas. It forms the inferior and lateral border of the suboccipital triangle. The superior oblique muscle attaches to the transverse process of the atlas and ascends posteriorly and medially to attach to the occiput, deep and lateral to the attachment of the semispinalis capitis muscle. The superior oblique muscle forms the superior and lateral borders of the suboccipital triangle.

When the fascia and fat are carefully removed from within the triangle formed by these muscles, several key structures become evident. The prominent vertebral artery is deep within the triangle (see Fig. 3–19). It courses in a lateral-to-medial direction across the triangle as it exits the transverse foramen of the first cervical vertebra and curves medially behind the lateral mass of the atlas in its path across the triangle. It then pierces the posterior atlanto-occipital membrane to turn cranially toward the foramen magnum and the brain stem, where it joins with the opposite vertebral artery to form the basilar artery.

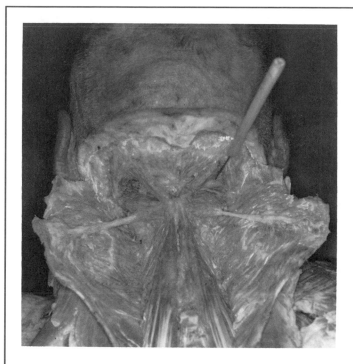

Figure 3–19. Suboccipital triangle.

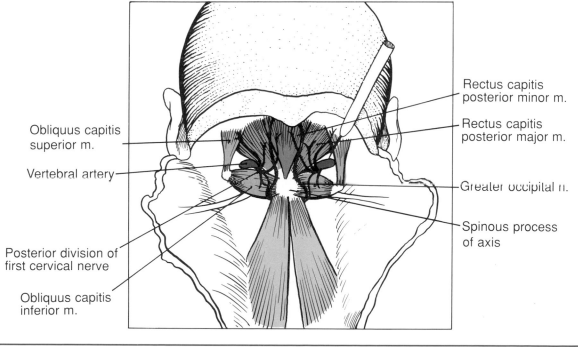

Obliquus capitis superior m.

Vertebral artery

Posterior division of first cervical nerve

Obliquus capitis inferior m.

Rectus capitis posterior minor m.

Rectus capitis posterior major m.

Greater occipital n.

Spinous process of axis

The dorsal ramus of the first cervical nerve, also known as the suboccipital nerve, is also located within the triangle, usually between the vertebral artery and the inferior oblique muscle. This nerve supplies the motor innervation to the four suboccipital muscles.

The second cervical dorsal ramus is a larger nerve and emerges from under the inferior oblique muscle. Therefore, it is not within the triangle but courses around the caudal border of the inferior oblique muscle. It divides into a medial and a lateral branch, with the medial branch forming the greater occipital nerve, which is an important sensory nerve, and the lateral branch supplying the splenius capitis, longissimus capitis, and semispinalis capitis (see Fig. 3–19). The lateral branch often is joined by the dorsal ramus of the third occipital nerve.

The suboccipital muscles are positioned to move the occiput-atlas-axis complex independently of the lower cervical spine. This function allows the lower cervical spine to be positioned and fixated while the upper cervical spine moves into positions that optimize the placement of the various sense organs of the head.

The inferior oblique muscle has a mechanically advantageous lever arm for rotation of the atlas on the axis, especially since its line of pull is posteriorly directed from the transverse process of the atlas toward the spinous process of the axis (Fig. 3–20). The lever arm is long because the transverse process of the atlas extends further laterally than any of the other cervical transverse processes, thereby placing it at a significant distance from the axis of motion for rotation. The rectus capitis posterior major has an excellent lever arm for occipital extension. Figure 3–19 shows the occipital attachment of the rectus capitis major and the superior oblique.

It is important to realize the depth of the suboccipital muscles and the tissues that overlie them. Pain in the suboccipital region often is attributed to involvement of the suboccipital muscles when in fact any of the overlying tissues may be involved. When palpating the suboccipital region in the area just lateral to the spinous process of the axis, the clinician should realize that from superficial to deep, the tissues include the skin, investing layer of fascia, and the trapezius, splenius capitis, semispinalis capitis, and suboccipital muscles.

SCALENE MUSCLES

The scalene muscles—anterior, middle, and posterior—serve several important functions for the cervical spine (Fig. 3–21). The anterior and middle scalene muscles border the neurovascular structures coursing through the thoracic outlet, and the position of the muscles typically results in the lower trunks of the brachial plexus and subclavian artery coursing between them (Fig. 3–22).

The scalene muscles are laterally placed and serve as important guys for the cervical spine in the frontal plane. Their line of force, however, is not limited to this plane. The anterior scalene muscle is attached to the first rib, usually by a prominent tendon, and courses upward and posteriorly to reach the anterior tubercles of the third through sixth cervical transverse processes. This anterior-to-posterior inclination provides a line of pull that is directed in the sagittal plane.

The term scalenus anticus syndrome is used to denote a potential cause of thoracic outlet syndrome. Neurovascular symptoms may result from compression of the subclavian artery and brachial plexus at the region of the anterior scalene as the

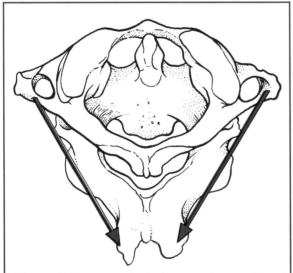

Figure 3–20. Mechanical advantage for rotation of the atlas on the axis by the inferior oblique muscle as it attaches to the transverse process of the atlas.

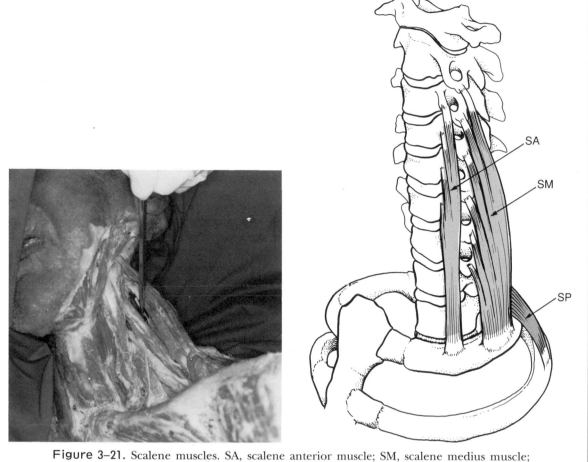

Figure 3–21. Scalene muscles. SA, scalene anterior muscle; SM, scalene medius muscle; SP, scalene posterior muscle. In left figure, the probe is placed between the left scalene medius and left levator scapulae muscles.

neurovascular bundle courses between the anterior and middle scalene muscles (see Fig. 3–22). This leads to sequelae such as edema and cyanosis in the arms and the inability to exercise or lift heavy objects. Irritation of the brachial plexus is thought to give rise to pain in the ulnar or median nerve distributions or into the shoulder and neck. The patient may complain of paresthesias or hyperesthesias after heavy exertion with the arms. Conservative treatment includes anti-inflammatory medication, exercises to condition muscles of the shoulder girdle, postural instruction, ergonomic interventions, and steroidal injections into the anterior scalene muscle.[15]

The middle scalene muscle also has an attachment to the first rib, but it is much broader than that of the anterior scalene muscle (see Fig. 3–21). Its posterior inclination is not as great as that of the anterior scalene muscle as it courses upward to attach to the anterior tubercles of the third through seventh cervical transverse processes. Its line of pull places it in an excellent position for dynamically stabilizing the cervical spine in the frontal plane.

The posterior scalene is attached to the second rib and courses upward and slightly anteriorly to attach to the posterior tubercles of the third through seventh cervical transverse processes.

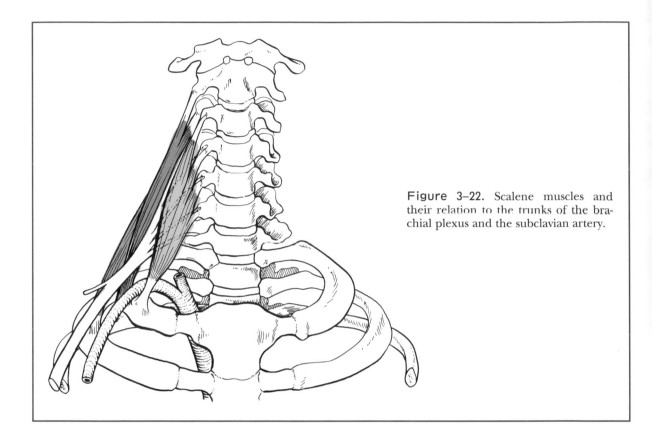

Figure 3–22. Scalene muscles and their relation to the trunks of the brachial plexus and the subclavian artery.

The posterior scalene crosses the first rib just behind the anterior scalene to reach the second (and sometimes the third) rib. Such a course places it immediately anterior to the levator scapulae muscle. Thus the anterior and posterior scalene muscles have different lines of force in the sagittal plane when compared with the posterior scalene because of their different attachments.

The action of the scalene muscles can be deduced from their attachments. They have a mechanically advantageous lever arm for lateral flexion of the cervical spine. The anterior scalene muscles working bilaterally can flex the cervical spine, but their lever arm is not as effective as that of the sternocleidomastoid muscle. Because they are cervical neck flexors, they also have the potential to sustain an acceleration injury.

The anterior scalene and levator scapulae muscles are oriented to provide an anterior-posterior line of pull over the cervical spine. Besides flexion and extension, such an orientation of the muscles helps to provide a check to anterior and posterior shear forces (Fig. 3–23). As noted above, the levator scapulae has a similar function to the deep erector spinae muscles (lumbar erector spinae) of the low back. The anterior scalene muscle is similar to the psoas major muscle in the lumbar spine in that both attach to the anterior aspect of vertebral transverse processes and course inferiorly and anteriorly from that point to reach their inferior attachment—the psoas major to the lesser trochanter and the anterior scalene to the first rib. The deep erector spinae and psoas major muscles are oriented to dynamically contribute to the control of anterior and posterior shear forces of the lumbar spine. Likewise, the levator scapulae and anterior scalene muscles are ideally positioned to have much the same mechanical effect on the cervical spine (see Fig. 3–23). Their respective attachments to the transverse processes help to provide sagittal plane stability of the cervical spine with much the same anterior-posterior reinforcing effect. Contraction of the levator scapulae muscle imparts a posterior

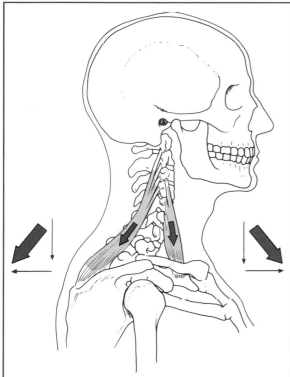

Figure 3–23. Stabilizing effect of the levator scapulae and anterior scalene muscles on the cervical spine. Such an arrangement offers stability of the cervical spine in the sagittal plane.

anterior tubercles of the cervical transverse processes and its upper part travels cranially and medially between the same anterior tubercles of the transverse processes to the atlas. A middle, more vertical part covers the cervical vertebral bodies. The longus capitis courses from the anterior tubercles of the cervical transverse processes to the base of the occiput (see Fig. 3–18).

Working alone, the muscles can act as flexors of the cervical spine. This motion is anterior sagittal rotation of the cervical vertebrae because the muscles are located anterior to the center of rotation for flexion and extension of the cervical spine. In addition, contraction of the muscles increases the compressive force between the cervical vertebrae. Their position on the anterior aspect of the cervical vertebrae renders them vulnerable to an acceleration injury, which results in a forced hyperextension motion of the cervical spine.

Hyperextension injuries to the cervical spine typically cause more soft tissue injury than any other forced motions because the range of forced cervical extension usually is greater than motion in any other direction. The forced hyperextension motion often damages the anterior structures of the neck because the violent cervical extension motion is not checked until the occiput comes into contact with the posterior aspect of the lower neck. In contrast, a forced flexion maneuver usually is stopped from reaching extreme ranges because the chin comes in contact with the upper portion of the sternum and further flexion is restrained. When a forced hyperextension motion is described by the patient, especially that occurring with a motor vehicle accident, the longus colli and capitis muscles should be suspected as possible sources of pain. In addition to being painful to palpation, injury to these muscles may cause difficulty in active anterior sagittal rotation of the cervical vertebrae. The patient may be unable to lift the weight of the head from the supine position.

It can be readily appreciated that nearly every aspect of the cervical vertebrae has muscular attachments, with all the processes and the vertebral bodies having various muscles attached to them. The gap between the right and left longus colli muscles on the anterior aspect of the cervical vertebrae is one of the few bony regions without muscle attachments. This region serves as an

shear force to the cervical spine; contraction of the anterior scalene muscle results in an anterior shear force.

ANTERIOR MUSCLES

Longus Colli and Capitis

The longus colli and capitis muscles cover the anterior aspect of the cervical vertebral bodies (Fig. 3–24). The course of the longus colli muscle is extensive because it extends between the upper thoracic vertebrae and the atlas. It is especially prominent because of the numerous tendon slips that arise from this muscle to attach to each cervical level. The longus colli muscle is triangular in that its lower portion travels cranially and laterally from the thoracic vertebral bodies to the

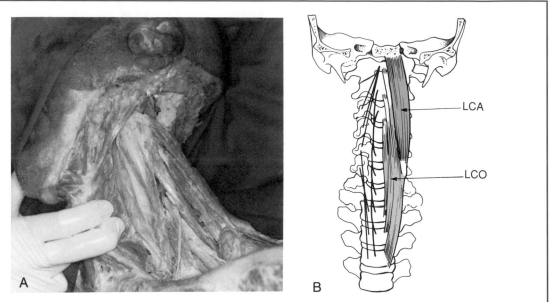

Figure 3–24. *A* and *B,* Longus colli and capitis muscles. LCA, longus capitis muscle; LCO, longus colli muscle.

important landmark during anterior surgical approaches to the cervical spine. The two longus colli muscles are immediately proximal to two important structures: the vertebral arteries and the cervical sympathetic chain.

Rectus Capitis Anterior and Lateralis

The rectus capitis anterior and lateralis muscles have a limited expanse, coursing from the anterior aspect of the atlas to the occiput. Although an action such as occipital flexion can be deduced from their location and lines of pull, it is also reasonable to consider these muscles as structures that contribute to proprioception for occipital motion rather than as prime movers. As mentioned already, and discussed further later, muscles that interlink the cervical spine have a dense array of muscle spindles. This important source of afferent input from the muscles provides the central nervous system with proprioceptive data that allow for continual adjustments of head and neck postural positioning.

Infrahyoid and Suprahyoid

The most superficial muscles of the anterior neck can be conveniently divided into those muscles inferior to the hyoid bone—the infrahyoid muscles—and those superior to the hyoid bone—the suprahyoid muscles. The infrahyoid muscles consist of the sternohyoid, sternothyroid, thyrohyoid, and omohyoid muscles. They are also referred to as the *strap muscles* and are covered by their own fascial complex (Fig. 3–25). These muscles act to fixate or depress the hyoid bone and thyroid cartilage. The suprahyoid muscles consist of the digastric, stylohyoid, mylohyoid, and geniohyoid muscles. These muscles fixate or elevate the hyoid bone. Fixation and cyclic movement of the hyoid bone are essential during deglutition, and thus, the actions of these muscles are important for the coordination of that activity.

When the hyoid bone is fixated, muscles attached to it can exert action on other movable segments. For example, with the hyoid bone stabilized, the digastric and mylohyoid muscles can depress the mandible and are especially active during swallowing and chewing. These subtle movements alternated with hyoid stabilization best illustrate the complex coordination between these muscles. As an example, the mylohyoid elevates the floor of the mouth during the initial stages of deglutition, and the geniohyoid acts to depress the mandible. The sternothyroid muscle acts to draw the larynx downward after it has been elevated, which is essentially a component of the cyclic activity of the larynx that normally occurs during swallowing or vocalization.

Although the action of the infrahyoids and suprahyoids is not fully understood, it is apparent that movements of the hyoid bone are coordinated with movements of the tongue to accommodate the various textures encountered during the ingestion of food and liquids. A precise, highly complex integration of the neuromuscular system essentially directs food from the oral cavity to the oral pharynx and on to the esophagus.

The infrahyoid and suprahyoid muscles also play an important role in head and neck posture. Postural positioning of the head and neck influences the state of resting muscle tension in mus-

cles related to the hyoid bone (Fig. 3–26). With a head and neck posture that results in the cervical spine being more forward in the sagittal plane and the occiput subsequently being placed in excessive extension to keep the eyes looking more horizontally instead of in a downward direction as a result of this forward cervical spine, a passive tensile force is imparted to the hyoid muscles. The increased tension of these muscles results in the mandible being depressed and translated posteriorly. To counteract this passive pull into mandibular depression, the patient must actively and continuously contract the temporalis and masseter muscles to keep the mouth closed.

Such excessive muscle activity of the primary muscles that close the mouth may result in myofascial pain related to the temporalis and masseter or discomfort in the temporomandibular joint. Referred pain from the temporalis also may take the form of a toothache complaint in the maxillary teeth. The clinician should recognize these biomechanical relationships between the face, jaw, and cervical spine, especially when the constellation of complaints include an excessively dry mouth (from being passively pulled

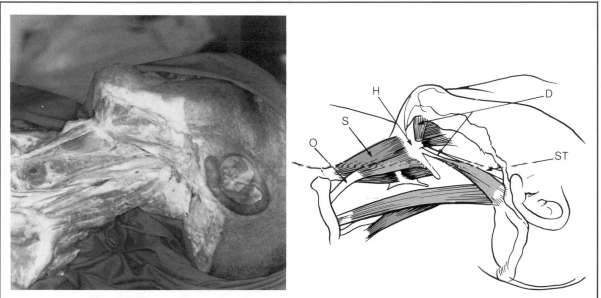

Figure 3–25. Infrahyoid muscles from an anterior view. D, anterior and posterior bellies of digastric muscle; H, hyoid bone; O, omohyoid muscle; S, sternohyoid muscle; ST, stylohyoid muscle.

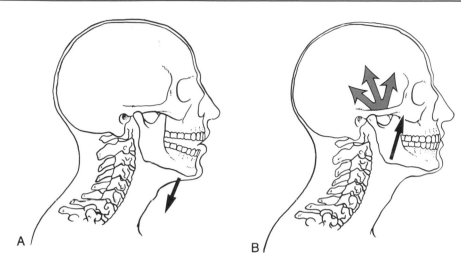

Figure 3–26. *A* and *B*, Relation between head and neck posture and the resultant contraction of the muscles of mastication (temporalis and masseter). Tightness of the anterior structures of the neck forces the mandible into an open position. Active and continuous contraction by the muscles of mastication is necessary to keep the mouth closed.

open and mouth breathing), difficulty swallowing, suboccipital headaches, teeth clenching, pain in the head and face over the temporal region, and tightness over the region of the throat.

MUSCLE RECEPTORS: CLINICAL IMPLICATIONS

Both the macroscopic and the microscopic structure of muscle have been previously detailed, which allowed the mechanical basis of motor activity related to the spine to be addressed.[12] Such a perspective is essential to more fully appreciate the function of muscle during activity and its role in dynamic stabilization rather than as a conglomerate of origins, insertions, and actions.

To meet the concurrent demands of stability and mobility, muscle function can be summarized by grouping muscle activity in the following manner (Table 3–2):

1. Agonist muscle—concentrically contracts and acts to accelerate the movable segment

2. Antagonist muscle—eccentrically contracts and acts to decelerate the movable segment

3. Synergist muscle—contracts isometrically and acts to stabilize a movable segment

The combination of motor activity controlling and regulating acceleration, deceleration, and stabilizing functions affords the spine the opportunity to meet the conflicting demands of mobility and stability.

In the low back, a strong case can be made for the importance of conditioning the neuromuscular system to optimize muscle performance, especially since increasing the stability of the lumbopelvic region is such an important clinical consideration. Treatment of the low back often is designed around the principle of increasing the strength and endurance of the low back musculature, especially the extensor muscles, to use the shock-absorbing and force-attenuating capabili-

Table 3–2. Muscle Function
Agonist—concentric—accelerator
Antagonist—eccentric—decelerator
Synergist—isometric—stabilizer

ties of the trunk and lower-extremity musculature.[2, 9] Therefore, the objective of treatment focusing on enhancing neuromuscular performance is an important one for low back pain patients.

When the structure and function of the cervical spine musculature are considered and viewed in concert with the unique relation between the cervical spine and the central nervous system, a slightly different focus emerges. This focus is one of movement facilitation in patients with cervical spine disorders and, secondarily, strength training. This different focus is due in part to the unique structural characteristics and functional demands of cervical spine musculature and the relation between the cervical spine muscles, movements of the cervical spine, and the sense organs of the head. Because reflex activity primarily helps to determine motor behavior of the muscles, a review of the receptor system in the muscle is helpful.

Muscles essentially have five types of receptors: muscle spindles, tendon organs, pacinian corpuscles, undifferentiated receptors that are essentially free nerve endings, and capsulated mechanoreceptors. For the purposes of this chapter, only the muscle spindles, tendon organs, and undifferentiated muscle receptors are considered.

Muscle Spindles

The density of receptor organs is not uniform in all muscles. For example, muscles spindles are found in much higher concentration in those muscles that control precise movements.[13] By way of comparison, the suboccipital muscles have about 150 to 200 muscle spindles per gram of muscle tissue, whereas the larger rectus femoris muscle contains 50 muscle spindles per gram of muscle tissue.

Some of the highest concentrations of muscle spindles per gram of muscle tissue are in the paraspinal muscles of the cervical region. Spindle density in the range of 200 to 500 spindles per gram of muscle tissue can be found in the deeper muscle fibers of the cervical spine, especially the muscles that attach at each segment rather than spanning several segments.[5] Muscle spindles are especially dense around the slow twitch or oxidative muscle fibers, which typically are considered the postural muscles related to the spine.

The structure of a muscle spindle can be succinctly summarized as a receptor consisting of the following (Fig. 3–27):

1. Several specialized muscle fibers
2. A connective tissue capsule filled with a ge-

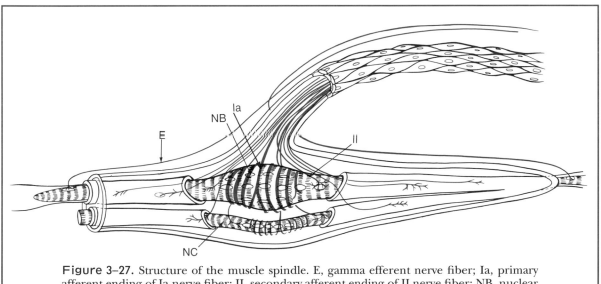

Figure 3–27. Structure of the muscle spindle. E, gamma efferent nerve fiber; Ia, primary afferent ending of Ia nerve fiber; II, secondary afferent ending of II nerve fiber; NB, nuclear bag fiber; NC, nuclear chain fiber.

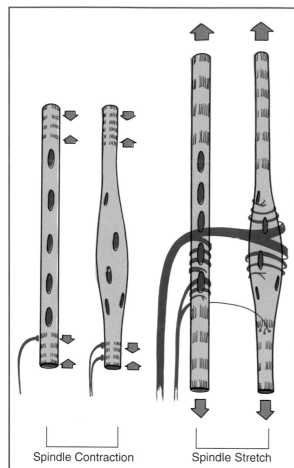

Spindle Contraction   Spindle Stretch

Figure 3-28. Two ways in which the central portion of the spindle can be elongated: stretch and fusimotor contraction. Passive stretch of the muscle elongates the central region of the spindle, and contraction of the end of the spindle causes a resultant stretch over the central region of the spindle.

latinous substance surrounding the middle portion of the muscle fibers

3. Afferent and efferent nerves leaving and entering the spindle

The efferent nerves to the muscle spindle terminate on the ends of the muscle spindle. This region corresponds to the striated portion of the muscle spindle. As a result of contraction of the ends of the spindle, the middle portion of the spindle becomes elongated. Elongation of

the middle portion can occur with any lengthening of the muscle, as, for example, the lengthening that occurs with stretch (Fig. 3-28).

The central region of the muscle spindle is the portion that can elongate because it is precisely this phenomenon that is sensed by the mechanoreceptive afferent nerve endings that ramify on this central region. The central region of the muscle spindle can, therefore, be elongated by one of two separate actions: contraction of the ends of the muscle spindle or stretch of the muscle, which will in turn stretch the spindle itself and distort the central region of the spindle.

Three types of muscle spindles commonly are described: bag 1, bag 2, and chain fibers. The terms bag and chain refer to the arrangement of nuclei within the muscle spindle and not to the shape of the spindle itself.

Afferent Nerve Supply

There are two anatomically and functionally distinct types of afferent nerves supplying the muscle spindles (see Fig. 3-27). The first type is the *primary ending*, which is essentially spiraled around the middle portion of the muscle spindle. The primary afferent ending innervates all fibers of the spindle—bag 1, bag 2, and chain fibers.

The *secondary ending* usually is also spiraled about the middle of the spindle but is adjacent to the primary ending on the chain fibers. The secondary afferent ending is not restricted to a spiral shape but can have nonspiral morphology that is referred to as flower spray ending. This ending is not restricted to the chain fibers and can terminate on chain or bag fibers, although it is primarily concerned with innervation of the chain fibers. Both the primary and the secondary endings provide the afferent input from the muscle spindles to the central nervous system.

Efferent Nerve Supply

Efferent axons (fusimotor axons) provide the efferent output from the central nervous system to the muscle spindle and terminate on the ends of the spindle. The bag 1 fiber typically receives an axon dedicated to that muscle spindle fiber only, whereas the bag 2 and chain fibers usually are innervated by branches of the same axon. Most of the cell bodies for these fusimotor axons reside in the ventral horn of the spinal cord. There are, however, a significant number of alpha motor neurons (those neurons that innervate the extrafusal fibers of skeletal muscle) that branch as they innervate the skeletal muscle fibers to also supply the muscle spindle. These unique efferent axons are called skeletofusimotor axons.

Functional Considerations

The afferent nerves are discharged whenever the length of the muscles is changed or whenever the rate of firing of the fusimotor axons is increased. Contraction of the fusimotor fibers has a negligible effect on total muscle force; however, contraction of the ends of the spindles elongates the middle of the spindle by about 20 per cent.[4] For the same degree of elongation to occur by way of muscle stretch in the central region of the spindle, the muscle would need to be lengthened to its physiological limit. Therefore, both muscle stretch and fusimotor activity have comparable effectiveness in initiating discharge from the afferent nerves of the spindle.[7]

There is a functional difference, however, between the results of fusimotor axon discharge of the bag 1 fiber and those of the bag 2 and chain fibers. When the bag 1 fiber is held at a constant length and the fusimotor axon discharges to initiate spindle contraction, the effect on afferent discharge from the spindle is not as pronounced as when the muscle is being simultaneously stretched while the ends of the muscle spindle are contracting.[3] This increase in afferent activity as a result of simultaneous spindle contraction and muscle lengthening is referred to as the dynamic role of the bag 1 spindle, with dynamic in this instance referring to the elongation of the spindle through stretch.

In contrast, bag 2 and chain fibers are referred to as static because contraction of the spindle ends results in an increase in the discharge rate of the afferent axons that supply the spindle, regardless of the spindle length. The dynamic component of the spindle system is an increase in spindle sensitivity while the spindle length is changing; the static component of the spindle system is an increase in afferent discharge of the spindle at all lengths.

These anatomical and functional differences result in the spindle having an exceptional sensitivity to muscle stretch. When the stretch is small, the primary afferent ending readily responds to the subtle change in muscle length. It is not necessarily the velocity or the extent of the stretch that elicits spindle activity but rather the motion.[8] This exquisite sensitivity to movement provides a reasonable explanation for the rapid adaptation of muscle contraction to postural changes. It also illustrates that even a small range of active or passive motion of the cervical spine has the potential to influence this mechanoreceptor system.

When stretching of the muscle is terminated and the muscle is held at a constant length for a period of time, the discharge rate diminishes. A new sensitivity of the spindle afferents is established at this new length, and the muscle spindle is once again sensitive to small changes in muscle lengths. This is perhaps the basis for treatment techniques for the spine that purport to reset the muscle spindle complex.

Tendon Organs

Tendon organs usually are restricted to the regions of the muscle tendon junction and are not typically located in the tendon proper. They primarily consist of collagen and associated nerve endings encased in a connective tissue capsule. The capsule of the tendon organ has a unique structure in that one end attaches to the collagen of the tendon and the opposite end is attached to the muscle fibers (Fig. 3–29).

Sensory axons enter the middle of the tendon organ capsule and course between the collagen strands. Such an arrangement allows for distortion of the axon terminals on deformation of the capsule. This distortion depolarizes the axon terminal and initiates an afferent volley from the tendon organ toward the central nervous system.

Because the muscle fibers attach directly into the tendon organ capsule, muscle contraction results in an immediate distortion of the axon terminals with a resultant increase in afferent nerve fiber activity. However, because the parallel arrangement of collagen within the tendon is especially resistant to stretching, passive stretch of the muscle (which passively lengthens muscle tissue but not the region of the tendon or the muscle-tendon junction) does little to initiate discharge of the sensory axons.

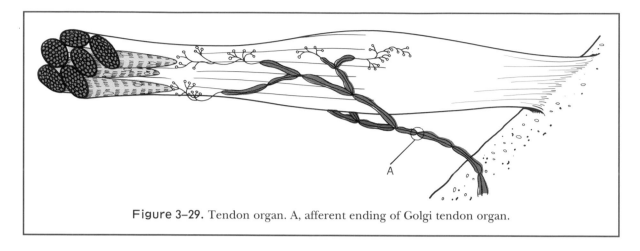

Figure 3–29. Tendon organ. A, afferent ending of Golgi tendon organ.

Contraction of a single muscle fiber has the potential to initiate discharge from the sensory nerve of the tendon organ to the central nervous system.[6] Therefore, it should be realized that the tendon organ is a low-threshold receptor, so that only a low contractile force of the muscle is necessary to initiate afferent discharge from the tendon organ. Another way of stating this is that the sensitivity of tendon organs to muscle force is comparable to the sensitivity of muscle spindles to muscle length.[7] The role of the tendon organs is to signal to the central nervous system moment-to-moment changes in force development of the muscle.

Undifferentiated Receptors

There are more undifferentiated receptors in the muscles than muscle spindles and tendon organs. Consequently, there are more afferent axons in muscle originating from undifferentiated receptors than axons originating from spindles or tendon organs. These undifferentiated receptors typically are supplied by afferent nerves of the type III and type IV classes, which makes the conduction velocity of these afferent nerves slower than that of the spindles and tendon organs. Undifferentiated receptors are distributed among all aspects of the muscle tissue with the exception of the capillary network and are essentially free nerve endings.[14]

The functions of this vast array of undifferentiated receptors have not been fully elucidated.

One primary function relevant to a discussion of the cervical spine appears to be nociception. Nociceptors typically are depolarized by thermal, mechanical, and chemical stresses. From the standpoint of cervical spine injuries, mechanical and chemical activation of the nociceptive system is important. Mechanical stresses are those stresses or combinations of stresses that result in the nociceptor being depolarized. Such stresses include tension or compression of sufficient magnitude to depolarize the receptor system. Chemical stresses refer to alterations in the chemical milieu resulting from tissue injury. This chemical environment, especially when combined with the hypoxic effects resulting from stasis, acts to depolarize the nociceptor.

SUMMARY

It is essential that the clinician have a three-dimensional appreciation of the muscles related to the cervical spine. Likewise, an understanding of the receptor system is important to provide a scientific rationale for many of the neuromuscular treatment approaches used in the management of mechanical neck pain.

Changes in the resting state of muscle tension are common with many cervical spine disorders that affect the intervertebral disc, apophyseal joints, nerve roots, and cervical spinal canal. Likewise, muscles themselves may be the source of patient complaints and often sustain acceleration injuries.

The primary goal of treatment in cervical spine problems is to reactivate the neck. This essentially means that treatment techniques should be designed around the principle of facilitating movement in a coordinated pattern of motion that minimizes stress to injured structures. Using active motion, contract-relax techniques, rhythmic stabilization, neuromuscular facilitation techniques, and passive joint and soft tissue mobilization, functional improvements become more attainable. With a three-dimensional appreciation of the anatomy and an understanding of the receptor system, the clinician is better able to optimize the healing environment of the injured tissues while promoting coordinated movement of the head and neck.

REFERENCES

1. Ashton-Miller JA, McGlashen KM, Herzenberg JE, Stohler CS: Cervical muscle myoelectric response to acute experimental sternocleidomastoid pain. Spine 15:1006–1012, 1990.
2. Biering-Sorenson F: Physical measurements as risk indicators for low back trouble over a one year period. Spine 9:106–119, 1984.
3. Boyd IA: The action of the three types of intrafusal fibers in isolated cat muscle spindles on the dynamic and length sensitivities of primary and secondary sensory endings. *In* Taylor A, Prochazka A (eds): Muscle Receptors and Movement. London, Macmillan, 1981, pp 17–32.
4. Boyd IA: The response of the fast and slow nuclear bag fibers and nuclear chain fibers in isolated cat muscle spindles to fusimotor stimulation, and the effect of intrafusal contraction on the sensory endings. QJ Exp Physiol 61:203–252, 1981.
5. Dvorak J, Dvorak V: Manual Medicine: Diagnostics. Thieme, New York, 1990, p 42.
6. Fukami Y, Wilkinson RS: Responses of isolated Golgi tendon organs of the cat. J Physiol (Lond) 265:673–689, 1977.
7. Hasan Z, Stuart D: Mammalian muscle receptors. *In* Davidoff R (ed): Handbook of the Spinal Cord. New York, Marcel Dekker, 1984, pp 560–567.
8. Houk JC, Rymer WZ, Crago PE: Dependence of dynamic response of spindle receptors on muscle length and velocity. J Neurophysiol 46:143–166, 1981.
9. Mayer TG, Smith SS, Keeley J, Mooney V: Quantification of lumbar function. Pt 2. Sagittal plane strength in chronic low back pain patients. Spine 10:765–772, 1985.
10. McNab I: Acceleration injuries of the cervical spine. J Bone Joint Surg [Am] 46:1797–1799, 1964.
11. Nolan JP, Sherk HH: Biomechanical evaluation of the extensor musculature of the cervical spine. Spine 13:9–11, 1988.
12. Porterfield JA, DeRosa C: Mechanical Low Back Pain: Perspectives in Functional Anatomy. Philadelphia, WB Saunders, 1992.
13. Richmond FJ, Abrahams VC: What are the proprioceptors of the neck? Prog Brain Res 50:245, 1979.
14. Stacey MJ: Free nerve endings in the skeletal muscle of the cat. J Anat 105:231–254, 1969.
15. Sherk HH, Uppal GS: Congenital bony anomalies of the cervical spine. *In* Frymoyer JW (ed): The Adult Human Spine. New York, Raven Press, 1992, pp 1015–1036.
16. Takebe K, Vitti M, Basmajian JV: The functions of semispinalis capitis and splenius capitis muscles: An electromyographic study. Anat Rec 179:477–480, 1974.
17. Travell JG, Simons DG: Myofascial Pain and Dysfunction. Baltimore, Williams & Wilkins, 1983, pp 183–189, 202–218.

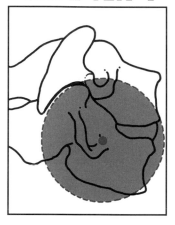

CHAPTER 4

ARTICULATIONS OF THE CERVICAL SPINE

Although certain anatomical features of the articulations in the cervical spine have similar counterparts in the thoracic and lumbar spine, there are several aspects that are unique to the cervical region. The unciform joints and the articulation between the dens of the axis with the atlas, for example, are highly specialized in both structure and function. In addition, the apophyseal, atlantoaxial, and atlanto-occipital joints as well as the intervertebral discs demonstrate distinct anatomical features that contribute to the unique biomechanics of the cervical spine.

The various articulations of the cervical spine conspicuously lack bony mass and serve discrete functions. It is apparent that the mass of the various articulations has been sacrificed in favor of increased mobility. The wide range of mobility in the cervical spine is of importance because this allows the key sensory organs such as the eyes and ears to be optimally positioned through an array of head and neck movements. By comparison, weight-bearing requirements for the articulations of the cervical spine stem largely from the necessity to absorb the compressive forces attributed to the weight of the head and the action of the muscles crossing the cervical spine (Fig. 4–1).

This chapter details the key anatomical components that contribute to the articulations of the cervical spine. From such a perspective, the functional anatomy of the articulations can be considered. Included is a look at the atypical vertebrae of the upper two segments, the cervical vertebrae of the lower cervical spine, the apophyseal joints and supporting ligaments, and the intervertebral disc.

There has been a paucity of research conducted in regard to the cervical spine as compared with that in regard to the lumbar spine. The clinician often extrapolates research from one area of the spine to explain phenomena in another area. In some instances, the information may be accurate, but in others, it has the potential to be misleading. Such broad generalizations regarding the articulations have been avoided as much as possible, but the importance of applying basic scientific knowledge from one spinal region to another to further our understanding is recognized.

The biomechanics of the cervical spine can be daunting to the clinician who deals with nonsurgical conditions. In most situations, however, these intricate mechanics can only be assessed

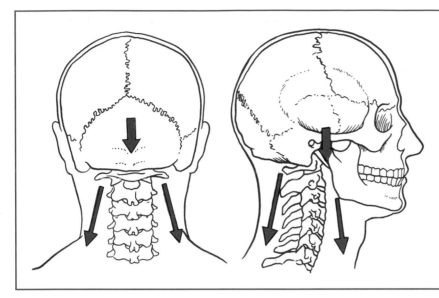

Figure 4-1. Compressive force is exerted on the cervical spine by muscle contraction and the weight of the head.

with sophisticated technology, and therefore, their clinical relevance is of questionable value. It is necessary to place these mechanics in proper perspective as much as possible. This chapter explains the mechanics in a practical rather than strictly academic manner. This allows the anatomical and biomechanical information of the articulations to be applied toward clinical practice.

BONY ANATOMY OF THE CERVICAL SPINE

When detailing the bones of the cervical column, it is convenient to divide the cervical spine into two anatomically and functionally distinct segments: the so-called lower cervical vertebrae, which include the third through the seventh cervical vertebrae, and the upper cervical spine, which includes the occiput, atlas (first cervical vertebrae), and axis (second cervical vertebra; (Fig. 4–2). The bony elements of the lower cervical spine, which is primarily concerned with the functional anatomy of the region below the second cervical vertebra, is described first. Because there are great similarities, both anatomically and functionally, between the lower cervical vertebrae

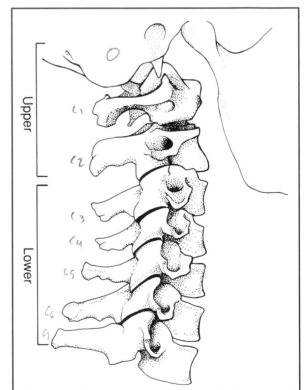

Figure 4-2. Functional divisions of the cervical spine: the upper cervical spine and the lower cervical spine.

and the upper thoracic vertebrae, it is clinically useful to consider this region as encompassing the cervicothoracic spine. For ease of discussion, this area is referred to here as the cervical spine.

Lower Cervical Spine

Vertebral Bodies

The body of a typical cervical vertebra in the lower cervical spine is elongated transversely, which results in the width being about 50 per cent greater than the anteroposterior diameter (Fig. 4–3). The cervical vertebral bodies are significantly smaller than the thoracic and lumbar vertebral bodies. As in the rest of the spine, the

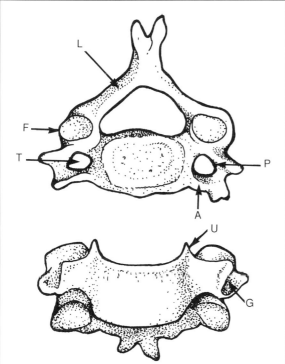

Figure 4–3. Bony elements of a typical cervical vertebrae. A, anterior component of transverse process; F, articular facet; G, gutter for nerve root; L, Lamina; P, posterior component of transverse process; T, transverse foramen; U, unciform process.

Table 4–1. Cervical Spine Muscle Attachments*
Anterior vertebral body
Longus colli
Spinous processes
Semispinalis thoracis and cervicis
Multifidus
Spinalis
Interspinales
Transverse processes—anterior tubercle
Scalene anterior
Longus capitis
Longus colli
Transverse processes—posterior tubercle
Splenius cervicis
Longissimus cervicis
Iliocostalis cervicis
Levator scapulae
Scalenus medius
Scalenus posterior
Anterior arch of the atlas
Longus colli
Lateral mass of the atlas
Rectus capitis anterior
Posterior arch of atlas
Rectus capitis posterior minor
Transverse process of the atlas
Rectus capitis lateralis
Superior oblique
Inferior oblique
Levator scapulae
Splenius cervicis
Scalenus medius
Spinous process of the axis
Inferior oblique
Rectus capitis posterior major
Semispinalis cervicis
Spinalis cervicis
Interspinalis
Multifidus

*The regions of the vertebrae that the muscles attach to are listed.

primary function of the vertebral body is to serve as a load-bearing structure for compressive forces.[35] In the cervical spine, the primary compressive forces are caused by the weight of the head and the contraction of the surrounding musculature. Table 4–1 lists the muscles attached to the various regions of the cervical vertebrae, which, by virtue of their attachments and fiber direction, exert a compressive force to the cervical spine on contraction.

Unciform Processes

The superior planar surfaces of the vertebral bodies of the lower cervical spine are modified because of the presence of unciform processes projecting upward from the posterolateral rims of the body (see Fig. 4–3). The unciform process consists of a ridge that courses anteriorly and posteriorly on the lateral rim of the vertebral body. The ridge is not strictly in the sagittal plane, but the posterior aspect has a slight medial curve. This bony configuration effectively converts a planar superior vertebral plateau to a modified concave superior surface. As a result of this concave profile, the inferior aspect of the vertebral body is slightly beveled in a way to allow for an articulation with the uncinate processes of the subjacent vertebrae. These articulations result in the formation of the uncovertebral joints, or joints of Luschka (Fig. 4–4).[30] Although there is some disagreement, it is generally held that these are not true synovial joints.[28, 50]

The vertebral body is further modified in that the anterior rim of the inferior surface of the vertebral body projects downward in front of the subjacent intervertebral disc. This bony projection and the unciform processes provide a unique encasement for the intervertebral disc. By comparison, the intervertebral disc of the lumbar spine is bordered by bone only on its superior and inferior surfaces.

The uncinate processes typically are absent at birth and develop between ages 6 and 9.[3] They reach their mature form at about 18 years of

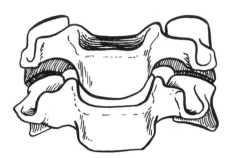

Figure 4–4. Uncovertebral joints. Note the curved orientation of the unciform processes and their location on the posterolateral rims.

age.[62] The first radiological manifestations of degenerative changes in the cervical spine occur at these uncovertebral joints.[53] Perhaps one of the reasons for this is that significant shear forces occur at these joints during flexion and extension of the cervical spine. Because the axis of motion in the cervical spine is located below the intervertebral disc, flexion and extension motion result in anterior and posterior shear forces, respectively, across the interface between the vertebral body and intervertebral disc and, therefore, between the articulating processes of the uncovertebral joints (Fig. 4–5). Shear forces potentially accelerate the degenerative changes in this region.

The orientation of the uncinate processes is

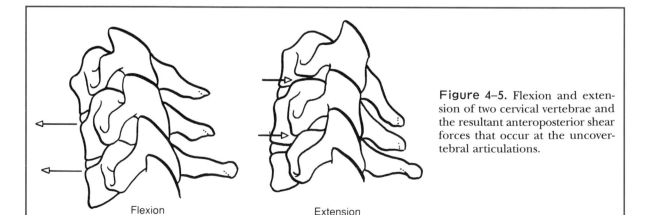

Figure 4–5. Flexion and extension of two cervical vertebrae and the resultant anteroposterior shear forces that occur at the uncovertebral articulations.

Flexion   Extension

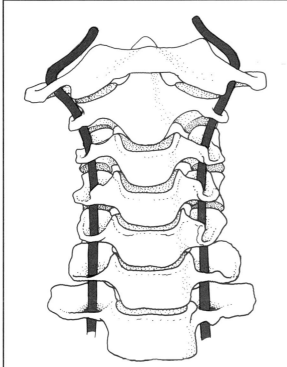

Figure 4–6. Cervical vertebrae with the vertebral artery in place. Lateral translation has the potential to compromise the vertebral artery.

also an effective means to minimize lateral motion between adjacent cervical vertebrae. This is especially relevant from a clinical standpoint. Because a lateral shear force that ultimately resulted in excessive lateral translation between adjacent vertebrae would quickly compromise the vertebral arteries in their course through the transverse foramen, it is essential that such motion be minimized (Fig. 4–6). The uncovertebral joints offer a bony block to lateral translation.

In summary, the uncovertebral joints are subject to the anterior and posterior shear forces that normally occur with flexion and extension of the cervical spine. However, they do not allow for lateral shear to occur, because this force tends to approximate or compress the beveled inferior edge of the vertebral body into the uncinate process of the subjacent vertebral body. The uncovertebral joints are discussed later in this chapter in the section on rotation of the cervical spine.

Pedicles

The pedicles project posterolaterally rather than directly posterior from the vertebral bodies in the cervical spine (see Fig. 4–3). As a result of a posterolateral orientation, the spinal canal is comparatively large and triangular rather than round. The size of the spinal canal is of importance because the vital medullary contents are housed here (see Chapter 2). The anterior wall of the spinal canal, which is formed in part by the posterior aspect of the vertebral bodies, is exceptionally straight.

Transverse Processes

The transverse processes are located on the sides of the vertebral body and the pedicles. Close inspection reveals an anterior component that projects laterally from the body and a posterior component that projects laterally from the pedicles. These projections are united at their lateral extent by a small strut of bone. The complete bony arrangement—the two lateral struts with their connection—is referred to as the transverse process.

Developmentally, the anterior component of this lateral projection is a rudimentary rib or costal process, and the posteriorly placed lateral projection is the true transverse process (Fig. 4–7). Therefore, the most precise anatomical term for this bony arrangement is costotransverse process, with the foramen formed by the bony strut connecting the two elements called the costotransverse foramen. Even though not anatomically accurate, the region usually is described simply as the transverse process, with the intervening foramen known as the transverse foramen.

The most lateral aspect of the rudimentary rib portion is referred to as the anterior tubercle of the transverse process. Although this is not precise in terms of anatomical terminology, it is a key clinical landmark. The anterior tubercle of the sixth cervical vertebra is particularly large and called the carotid tubercle. In this region, the common carotid artery, which is immediately anterior to the tubercle, can be compressed.

The true transverse process ends posteriorly as the posterior tubercle of the transverse process. As previously mentioned, even though the anterior (rudimentary rib) and posterior (true transverse process) elements fuse laterally, a space re-

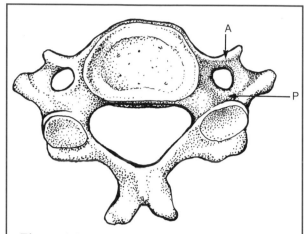

Figure 4–7. Components of the transverse process: the anterior and posterior tubercles with intervening transverse foramen. The anterior projection is the rudimentary rib or costal process and the posterior projection is the true transverse process. A, anterior component of transverse process; P, posterior component of transverse process.

mains medially that is the transverse foramen, through which the vertebral artery courses.

The true transverse process features a groove on its superior surface over which the spinal nerve of the cervical spine segment passes (Fig. 4–8). Note the difference between the course of the nerve roots and spinal nerves in the lumbar

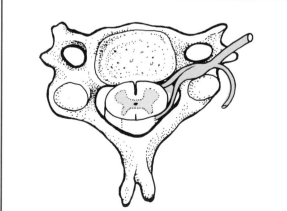

Figure 4–8. Superior view of cervical vertebrae showing how the cervical nerves exit over the superior groove.

spine and that in the cervical spine. In the lumbar spine, the lumbar roots curve around the *inferior* border of the pedicles of the upper vertebrae of the two adjacent vertebrae composing the motion segment, whereas in the cervical spine, the roots course over the *superior* border of the pedicles and then slope laterally and inferiorly along the upper surface of the transverse process. Further discussion of the paths and features of the cervical nerve roots and spinal nerves is found in Chapter 2.

The transverse processes serve as bony levers for the attachments of several muscles (see Table 4–1). The more laterally placed the attachment of the muscle to the transverse process, the longer the lever arm from the axis of cervical spine motion. Muscles attached to the transverse processes can exert forces that affect the horizontal, sagittal, and frontal plane positions of the cervical vertebrae in addition to increasing the compressive forces between the adjacent cervical vertebrae (see Chapter 3).

Spinous Processes

The spinous processes of the lower cervical spine are relatively short and feature bifid tips. They increase in length between the third cervical vertebra and the first or second thoracic vertebra. Because the spinous process serves as a prominent point of attachment for many cervical muscles, an effective lever arm is created owing to the length from the tip of the spinous process to the axis of rotation in each cervical segment (see Table 4–1).

A balance between lever arm length and spinous process length is essential to assure that the large range of motion available to the cervical spine is not compromised. If the spinous processes were excessively long, approximation of the bony tips would quickly occur during cervical extension. Even though the lever arm would have an increased length with elongated spinous processes, such an anatomical configuration would partially negate lever arm advantage. One of the bony adaptations that has been made to minimize this early bony approximation is the development of bifid spinous processes. Instead of quickly abutting into one another, the bifid processes seat into one another during extension, which allows a greater range of motion than would otherwise be possible.[35]

The significance of the spinous processes as levers for the muscles is demonstrated by the clinical condition known as clay shoveler's fracture. The mechanism of injury is described as one that occurs in a detrained, unconditioned worker who attempts to lift a full shovel of heavy clay or other material. The muscular forces that are transmitted to the spinous processes ultimately cause an avulsion-type fracture. The fracture is thought to be due to either excessive loading of the spinous processes by way of the forces of muscle contraction for an extended period, resulting in a fatigue fracture, or a single traumatic episode.[62] Gershon-Cohen and co-workers suggest that avulsion fracture of the spinous processes also can occur with hyperextension-hyperflexion whiplash injuries.[22] The mechanism suggested in these instances, however, is pull of the ligamentum nuchae on the spinous processes as a result of the hyperflexion motion of an acceleration injury.

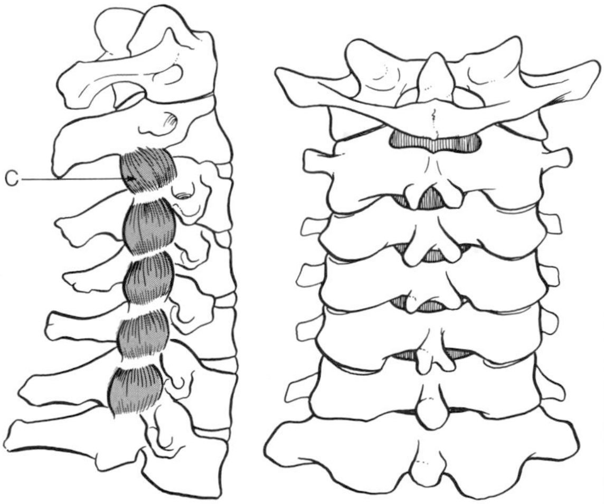

Figure 4–9. Apophyseal joints. C, apophyseal joint capsule.

Apophyseal Joints

One of the primary reasons for understanding the structure and function of the apophyseal joints is their potential contribution to painful neck syndromes. Although this statement may appear to be intuitively obvious, little objective data has been published in support of a facet syndrome in the cervical spine. Instead, inferences that the cervical apophyseal joints can be a source of pain have occurred on the basis of classic works published regarding the joints of the lumbar spine.[41, 45, 46] That the cervical spine apophyseal joints can be shown experimentally to be a source of pain has occurred with the works of several authors.[1, 5, 6, 18] In addition, the concept of pain referred from diseases or injuries of the cervical apophyseal joints must be considered. This section synthesizes the current understanding of these important joints to allow the clinician to develop evaluation and treatment procedures based on sound anatomy and mechanics. Later in the chapter, pain patterns stemming from the apophyseal joints are discussed.

As previously noted, there are distinct differences between the bones of the lower cervical spine and those of the upper cervical spine. Because of these differences, it is convenient to discuss the joints based on the same division into lower and upper elements. In some respects, the

joints between the second and third cervical vertebrae can be considered the transitional region between the upper and lower cervical spine. The joints of the lower cervical spine are reviewed first.

Each cervical vertebra in the lower cervical spine has four articular processes that can be subdivided into two superior articular processes and two inferior articular processes (Fig. 4–9). Each articular process has a facet surface lined with articular cartilage. The superior and inferior articular processes form an articular pillar that is prominent laterally at the junction of the pedicle and lamina. The cervical apophyseal joints are palpated as small domes through the overlying trapezius and deeper cervical muscles about 2 cm lateral to the spinous processes.

The mean inclination of the cervical facets in the lower cervical spine is about 45 degrees to the frontal plane, although this inclination increases slightly in the more caudal cervical vertebrae (Fig. 4–10).[40] The superior facets of the cervical vertebrae face posterior and superior and the inferior facets face anterior and inferior.

The joint capsules that connect the articular processes bearing the hyaline cartilage facets permit great mobility because of their relative laxity when compared with other connective tissue

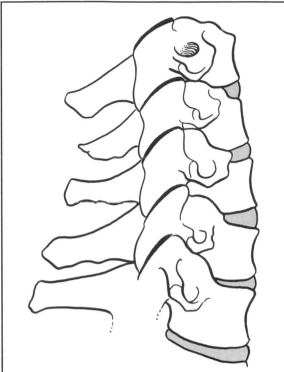

Figure 4–10. Planes of the cervical facets. The oblique plane tends to be more horizontal in the upper part of the cervical spine and more vertical in the lower part of the cervical spine.

Table 4–2. Lower Cervical Spine Range of Motion—Total Flexion and Extension

	Dvorak et al[15]	White & Panjabi[62]	Penning[53]
C2–3	10	8	12
C3–4	15	13	18
C4–5	19	12	20
C5–6	20	17	20
C6–7	19	16	15
C7–T1		6	

4–5). This translation measures about 2 to 3.5 mm. In general, there is slightly more anterior translation (1.9 mm) compared with posterior translation (1.6 mm). The two translations—1.9 and 1.6—when added together, provide for the upper limit of 3.5 mm.[52, 60]

The plane of the facets is one of the primary restraints to the anterior shear that occurs with flexion of the cervical spine. The uncinate processes that jut upward from the lateral aspect of the superior vertebral end plate provide a type of guide rail for this sagittal plane motion.[40] There is little evidence that a decrease in this translation can be assessed by palpation of segmental motion testing. More important, the reliability among examiners using such manual assessment techniques would necessarily be poor because of the small range of movement.

Of the segments caudal to C2, the C5-6 articulation is considered to have the greatest range of motion, and the C2-3 segment is considered to have the least (Table 4–2). It has been suggested that the increased incidence of spondylosis at the C5-6 level is due to the large range of motion available.[63] Boden and associates found that the level between C5 and C6 was the level most frequently considered abnormal in magnetic resonance scans of the cervical spine in asymptomatic subjects.[2] Thus, the imaging study must be correlated to signs and symptoms to determine whether age-related changes or the degenerative process has any bearing on the painful syndrome.

During flexion of the cervical spine, the upper cervical vertebra of the functional unit tilts and slides forward over the subjacent vertebra (Fig. 4–11).[40] This results in the inferior facet of the superior vertebra of the functional unit sliding superiorly and anteriorly over the superior facet of the inferior vertebra. In addition, flexion re-

structures in the body. As in the lumbar spine, meniscoid-like synovial folds have been described within the cervical apophyseal joints, but little is known about their role in function or pathology.[55] To develop an appreciation of apophyseal joint mechanics, they are described in reference to the flexion-extension motions of the lower cervical spine and then the coupled motions of rotation and lateral flexion.

Movement Patterns

Flexion and Extension. Flexion and extension of the lower cervical spine occurs in the sagittal plane. In the cervical segments caudal to C2, the motion is coupled. During flexion, an anterior translation of the vertebrae results, and during extension, a posterior translation occurs (see Fig.

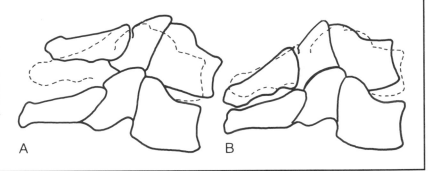

Figure 4–11. *A*, Tilt and anterior shear of the cervical vertebrae during flexion. *B*, Extension, which decreases the sagittal diameter of the canal because of the retrolisthesis that occurs.

A   B

sults in a compression of the anterior aspect of the disc, and the tilt results in a tensile force being imparted to the posterior aspect. Consequently, the cervical spinous processes become separated compared with the nonflexed position.

It is generally agreed that the tilt, which is essentially anterior sagittal rotation of the vertebrae, and the slide, which is a translation, occur simultaneously. Jones, however, has suggested that the slide follows the tilt.[32]

The pattern of vertebral motion in extension is reversed, with the inferior facets sliding downward and backward over the superior facets. More important, extension results in a decrease in the sagittal diameter of the vertebral canal of the cervical spine.[55] A slight retrolisthesis normally occurs as the upper vertebra of the motion segment translates posteriorly toward the spinal cord, which accounts for the posterior translation noted above (see Fig. 4–11). In contrast to the lumbar spine, little bulge of the annulus fibrosus of the intervertebral disc occurs during extension of the cervical spine. Instead, the retrolisthesis of the vertebra results in a shingling effect when the upper vertebra of the motion segment is compared with the lower vertebra.[55]

The center of rotation for flexion and extension in the cervical spine is different than in other areas of the spine.[40] Whereas the center of rotation in the lumbar spine is considered to be located within the intervertebral disc, the center of motion in the cervical spine is placed in the body of the subjacent vertebra (Fig. 4–12). When the location of this center of rotation is recognized, the upward and anterior glide of the inferior facet on the superior facet can be better appreciated because that motion is in fact a small arc of a circle whose center would be this axis of

motion. The radii of curvature formed as rotation and translation occur in the sagittal plane during flexion is not the same at all segments. A flatter arc is present in the upper cervical spine, and a more acute arc occurs at the more caudal cervical segments.[40] This change in rate of curvature of the arc in moving caudally probably is due to the gradual increase in facet plane incline in moving from the cephalad to caudal aspect of the cervical spine.

The center of rotation of the cervical spine segments below C2 can be appreciated from another important perspective. Recall that the vertebral arteries course through the transverse foramen. The transverse foramina are in proximity to the theoretical center of rotation of the cervical spine. This proximity is an important functional adaptation because it means that the ver-

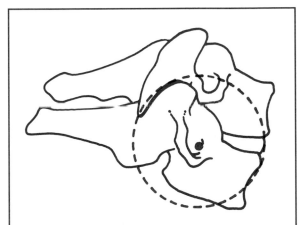

Figure 4–12. Location of the axis of motion for the cervical spine. Note how the arc of motion follows the plane of the facets.

tebral arteries undergo a small deformation as the spine moves from flexion to extension or vice versa. Were the location of the vertebral arteries to be significantly anterior or posterior to the center of cervical spine motion, more deformation of these vital arteries would be required the further they were located from the axis of motion.

The biomechanics of flexion and extension of the lower cervical spine segments can be applied to passive joint mobilization maneuvers. With the cervical spine in the neutral position, an anterior shear force applied by the clinician (often called an anterior glide) would be more effective in causing anterior translation at the C3-4 junction than at the C7-T1 articulation. This is because the facet planes have a more horizontal profile in the upper cervical regions and a resultant flatter arc of motion than the lower cervical spine. In comparison, to most effectively apply a passive joint mobilization maneuver that attempts to slide the inferior facet upward and anteriorly on the superior facet, a traction force concurrent with the anterior glide is used for the most caudal aspect of the lower cervical spine.

Table 4–2 provides useful information regarding segmental range of motion. There is a wide range of variability between studies, although trends can be noted. Such variability suggests caution when attempting to interpret segmental range of motion through palpation and raises the question as to whether such variability between individuals precludes useful information being gained. It is important to remember that the values given for flexion and extension ranges of motion are *total* ranges of sagittal motion. Assessments of hypomobility in flexion at one particular segment, for example, would be a difficult assessment with questionable reliability and reproducibility. What appears to be more useful is the recognition of a pain pattern that might occur with the application of a flexion or extension force during the assessment (see Chapter 5).

The complete spine has more stiffness (defined as resistance to deformation) in extension than in flexion. This implies that the spine is more flexible in flexion than in extension.[62] The increased flexibility is most apparent in the cervical and lumbar regions. When the posterior elements are experimentally removed, there is a resultant increase in extension but not flexion. This implies that the posterior joint complex plays a significant role in limiting extension but not flexion.[48, 62]

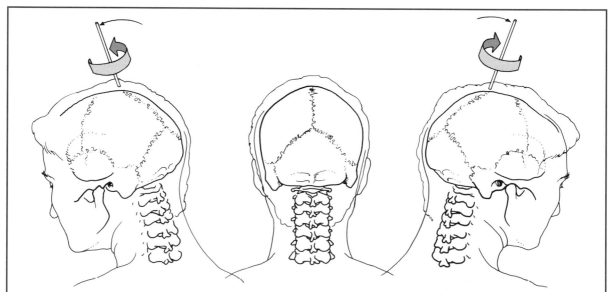

Figure 4–13. Coupled motion of lateral flexion and rotation. The action of rotation and lateral flexion is most strongly coupled in the cervical spine and less strongly coupled in the thoracic and lumbar spine.

Lateral Flexion and Rotation. In the cervical segments caudal to C2, the coupling patterns between lateral flexion and rotation are even more dramatic than those between flexion and translation. The coupling pattern results in lateral bending and rotation occurring in an ipsilateral direction (Fig. 4–13). If the cervical spine is laterally bent, the spinous processes of the vertebrae are directed toward the side of the convexity of the curve because of the obligatory vertebral rotation. For example, if the cervical spine is laterally bent to the right, there will also be a concurrent rotation of the vertebral body of the cervical vertebrae to the right.[33] The segmental lateral flexion and rotation capabilities for the lower cervical spine are listed in Tables 4–3 and 4–4.

The rotation–lateral flexion coupling patterns usually are described as being due to the plane of the facets that form the apophyseal joints. The coupling patterns, however, are probably due to the combined mechanics of the apophyseal joints and uncovertebral joints.[54] The shape of the uncinate processes located on the posterolateral rim of the vertebral body is such that their inner surfaces have a rounded, concave profile. The inner aspect of the uncinate process resembles an arc of a circle around which the superior vertebrae of the motion segment pivots (see Fig. 4–4).[54]

Aside from the articulation between the atlas and axis, the midcervical region displays the largest amount of rotation (see Table 4–4). The amount of axial rotation that is coupled with lateral flexion is not uniform at each level of the cervical spine, however. In general, there is a decrease in the amount of axial rotation associated with lateral bending when the upper cervical segments are compared with the lower ones.[62] This is probably due to the gradual change in horizontal inclination of the facets caudally. As the facets gradually approach the horizontal plane, more rotation is possible. Conversely, when the facets increase their frontal plane profile, rotation becomes more limited (Fig. 4–14). The increased frontal plane orientation of the lowest cervical vertebral facets minimizes the amount of rotation.

There is no correlation between a reduction in the range of motion and increasing degeneration. This is true for any direction of motion as well as total motion of the cervical spine. Perhaps most important from the clinical perspective, there is a large individual variation in range and

Table 4–3. Lower Cervical Spine Range of Motion—Lateral Bending in One Direction

	White & Panjabi[62]	Penning[53]	Moroney et al[48]
C2–3	10	6	4.7
C3–4	11	6	4.7
C4–5	11	6	4.7
C5–6	8	6	4.7
C6–7	7	6	4.7
C7–T1	4	6	4.7

Table 4–4. Lower Cervical Spine Range of Motion—Rotation in One Direction

	White & Panjabi[62]	Penning[53]	Dvorak et al[15]
C2–3	9	3	3
C3–4	11	6.5	6.5
C4–5	12	6.8	6.7
C5–6	10	6.9	7.0
C6–7	9	5.4	5.4
C7–T1	8	2.1	2.1

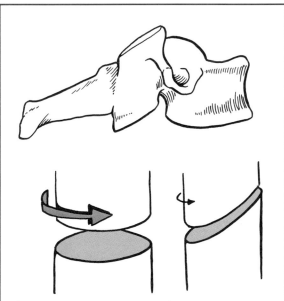

Figure 4–14. Plane of the apophyseal joints. Note how a more horizontal profile of the facet is conducive to rotation and a more frontal orientation precludes rotation.

distribution of rotational mobility in the lower cervical spine.[54] This statement is of great importance in regard to assessments of hypermobility or hypomobility of the cervical spine during passive motion testing. The range of segmental motion assessed during passive motion testing is perhaps not as critical as whether such motion testing reproduces familiar pain.

From the clinical perspective, a functional unit of the spine often is considered to be two vertebrae with the intervening disc and attached soft tissue. The motion of the facets of the superior vertebra on the subjacent vertebra of the functional unit can be compared to the wings of an airplane banking a turn. When the cervical spine is rotated to the right, the inferior facet on the right glides inferiorly and posteriorly on its articulating partner, and the inferior facet on the left glides superiorly and anteriorly. These mechanics of the functional spinal unit are considered important when selecting passive joint mobilization maneuvers to treat motion dysfunction of the cervical spine that contributes to the painful syndrome. To facilitate cervical rotation toward the right, a posterior- and downward-directed force on the right side or an upward- and anterior-directed force on the left matches the joint mechanics.

Upper Cervical Spine—Occipito-Atlanto-Axial Segment

Atlas

Although each component of the upper cervical spine is discussed separately, the occipito-atlanto-axial segment is actually a single functional unit with a distinct embryology and anatomy.[56] The understanding of the functional anatomy of this key region is enhanced when the major components are first discussed as separate entities.

The first cervical vertebra, the atlas, lacks a vertebral body (Fig. 4–15). In its place resides the superior projection from the second cervical vertebra, the dens, also known as the odontoid process. During embryological development, the vertebral body of the first cervical vertebra is "absorbed" into the vertebral body of the second cervical vertebra, forming the dens. Lacking a distinct vertebral body, the atlas resembles a washer set between the occiput and the axis. Act-

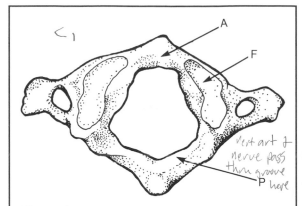

Figure 4–15. Bony elements of the atlas. A, anterior arch of the atlas; F, facet for occipital condyles; P, posterior arch of the atlas.

ing like a bearing, the atlas is thus positioned between the remaining cervical spine and the occipital condyles.

The major bony regions of the atlas are the anterior arch, the lateral masses, and the longer curved posterior arch (see Fig. 4–15). The anterior arch of the atlas merges into two lateral masses. On the superior aspect of these lateral masses are the large, kidney-shaped, concave articular facets for the occipital condyles. These superior articular facets face superiorly, with the anterior region of the facet directed medially. On the inferior aspect of the lateral masses are the flat-to-convex inferior articular facets, which articulate with the superior facets of the axis. Attached to the edges of the superior and inferior facets are the loose articular joint capsules for their respective joints.

The posterior arch is much larger than the anterior arch and accounts for about two-fifths of the complete ring of the atlas.[64] On the superior surface of the right and left sides of the posterior arch, a distinct groove identifies the bony channel over which the vertebral artery passes. Within this wide groove is also found the first cervical spinal nerve, which is the cervical dorsal ramus known as the suboccipital nerve. This nerve innervates the rectus capitis posterior major and minor, superior and inferior oblique, and semispinalis capitis muscles.[65] The bony groove is immediately posterior to the lateral mass of the atlas.

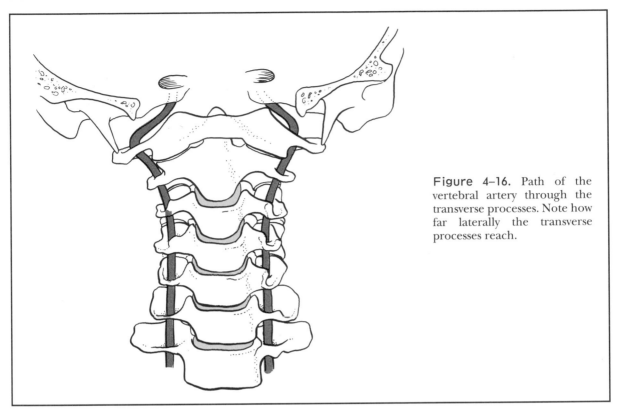

Figure 4–16. Path of the vertebral artery through the transverse processes. Note how far laterally the transverse processes reach.

The atlas has the widest profile of nearly all the cervical vertebrae because of the prominent transverse processes associated with it (Fig 4–16). The lateral extent of these elongated processes can be appreciated because they can be easily palpated through the skin of the lateral aspect of the neck in the region just posterior to the angle of the mandible. The length of these transverse processes affords the muscles attaching to them an optimal lever arm length for rotation of the atlas with its attached occiput (Fig. 4–17). The transverse processes thus serve as an excellent lever for the muscles (see Table 4–1).

On the inner aspect of the right and left sides of the anterior arch, two bony tubercles are present. From these tubercles arise the transverse ligament of the cruciate ligament complex (described below), which courses posteriorly to the upwardly projecting dens of the axis. This ligament is of key importance in maintaining the bony relation between the atlas and the axis and in preventing compression of the spinal cord by the dens.

Fractures of the atlas account for 25 per cent of all injuries to the C1-2 complex.[37] Several types of fractures are described. Fracture of the posterior arch is believed to result from cervical hyperextension and compressive loading that impinges the arch of the atlas between the occiput and the

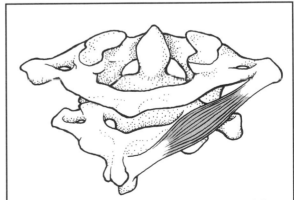

Figure 4–17. Attachment of the inferior oblique muscle. Note how its attachment to the most lateral aspect of the transverse process affords it an optimal lever arm for rotation.

large spinous process of the axis.[61] Other types of atlas fracture are the lateral mass fracture and the more widely recognized Jefferson fracture. A Jefferson fracture is considered a bursting fracture because of axial load being applied through the condyles of the base of the skull to the lateral masses. The force results in a lateral bursting of the atlas ring in tension and lateral displacement of the masses.[38] The frequency and potential for such fractures are mentioned to remind the clinician to maintain a high index of suspicion when the mechanics of injury described by the patient are consistent with the known mechanics of atlas fractures.

Axis

The axis is essentially the pivot on which the combined atlas and occiput rotate. On the superior surface of the vertebral body, the dens projects superiorly (Fig. 4–18). The anterior aspect of the dens contains a small articular facet that articulates with a facet located on the posterior surface of the anterior arch of the atlas. The posterior aspect of the dens has a grooved or slightly buckled appearance because of the presence of the transverse ligament. The apical ligament is attached at the tip of the dens, and the strong

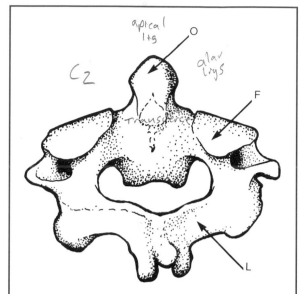

Figure 4–18. Bony elements of the axis. F, facet surface for articulation with atlas; L, lamina; O, odontoid process.

alar ligaments are attached to the sides of the dens. From a functional standpoint, the dens of the axis can be considered to reach up into the upper cervical spine region and attach to the oc-

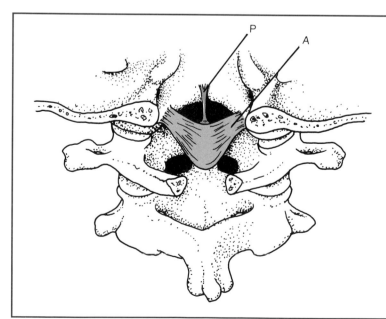

Figure 4–19. Attachments of the alar and apical ligaments. A, alar ligament; P, apical ligament.

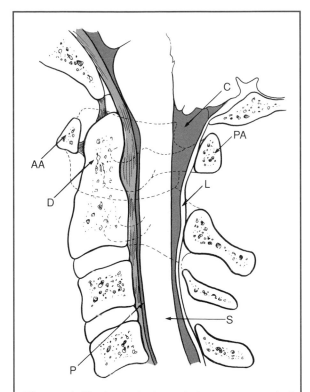

Figure 4-20. Sagittal view of the upper cervical spine showing how the dens abuts the lower portion of the brain stem. The cisterna magna helps to accommodate the translational movements. C, cisterna magna; D, dens; L, ligamentum flavum; P, posterior longitudinal ligament; PA, posterior arch of the atlas; S, spinal cord.

Diseases that weaken the connective tissue of the transverse ligament, such as rheumatoid arthritis, have the potential to compromise the spinal cord because of the instability that occurs between the atlas and axis. Therefore, caution should be exercised when using manual techniques for the upper cervical spine with such pathological conditions, and in many instances, such techniques are contraindicated.

When the axis is viewed from above, the large oval superior facets that articulate with the atlas can be seen immediately lateral to the dens. In comparison with the lower cervical spine, the superior and inferior facets of the axis do not form an articular pillar; instead, the superior facets are positioned well anterior to the inferior facets.

The lamina of the axis is the thickest of all cervical vertebrae.[64] In some regards, this lamina can be considered a transition point for the ligamentum flavum. The ligamentum flavum courses inferiorly toward the lamina of the third cervical vertebra. Above the level of the C2 lamina, the ligamentum flavum is renamed the posterior atlanto-axial membrane for the portion spanning C2 upward to C1 and the atlanto-occipital membrane for that portion spanning C1 to the occiput (Fig. 4-21).[62]

The right and left laminae of the axis are fused posteriorly with the large and thick spinous process. The prominence of the laminae is functionally significant because the strong pull of the muscles attached to the spinous process are transmitted through the laminae to the anterior aspect of the axis.

Special mention of the spinous process of C2 is warranted. This is one of the largest spinous processes in the cervical spine because it serves as a central point of attachment for several muscles (see Table 4-1). When the skin, fascia, and superficial muscles such as the trapezius and rhomboids are removed from the spine, it can be clearly seen that deeper muscles from the lower cervical and upper thoracic spine—most notably the large semispinalis cervicis complex—cross multiple segments and have a major attachment to the inferior aspect of the C2 spinous process; the muscles of the upper cervical spine, such as the inferior oblique and rectus capitis posterior major, attach to the same spinous process and course superiorly toward the C1 vertebra and the occiput. This muscular arrangement points out

cipital condyles by means of strong occipito-odontoid ligaments, in particular the alar ligaments (Fig. 4-19).

The importance of the transverse ligament in maintaining the position of the dens has already been noted. The intimate relation of the dens with the medullary tissues in the spinal canal is important to recognize. The posterior tip of the dens abuts the anterior aspect of the lowest portion of the brain stem and the upper spinal cord.[55] The presence of the large cisterna magna immediately posterior to the pons and medulla allows a space to accommodate the translatory movement of these vital neural tissues when the dens pushes them posteriorly during spinal movements (Fig. 4-20).

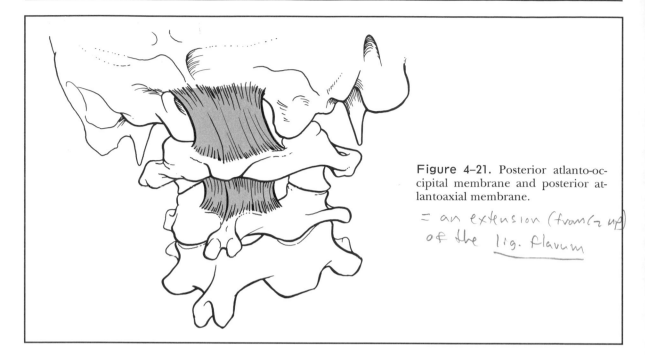

Figure 4–21. Posterior atlanto-occipital membrane and posterior atlantoaxial membrane.

= an extension (from C₂ up) of the lig. flavum

the important transitional position that the second cervical vertebra serves. Whereas many lower cervical segments are activated simultaneously with muscle contraction, the upper cervical spine retains the ability to carry out specific movements independent of the lower cervical spine because of this arrangement.[54]

Upper Cervical Joints

Motion between the occiput and atlas and between the atlas and axis is complex because of the uniqueness of the joints involved. Several synovial joints are present: between the occipital condyles and the lateral masses of the atlas, between the lateral masses of the atlas and axis, and between the anterior arch of the atlas and the odontoid process. Another synovial joint occurs between the transverse ligament of the cruciate ligament complex and the dens. No intervertebral discs are present between the atlanto-occipital and atlanto-axial articulations.

The configuration of the condylar surfaces of the occiput and atlas provides only minimal bony stability.[22] The atlanto-axial articulation also lacks bony congruency and, hence, inherent stability

(Fig. 4–22). Motion is controlled by the ligamentous and muscular network, and the absence of intervertebral discs, coupled with the reliance on the ligamentous framework to provide stability, renders this region particularly vulnerable to instability resulting from diseases that affect connective tissue, such as rheumatoid arthritis. Rheu-

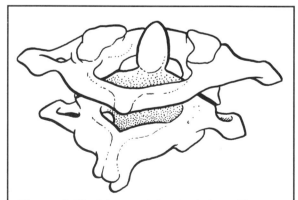

Figure 4–22. Atlanto-axial articulations. These articulations include those between the facets of the atlas and axis, the transverse ligament and dens, and the dens and anterior arch of the atlas.

matoid arthritis is well known to have the potential to result in atlanto-axial dislocation and upward migration of the dens.[47] Such excessive motion usually is prevented by the ligaments and joint capsules. To better describe the mechanics of the upper cervical spine, the component motions are analyzed as they were in describing the lower cervical spine.

Movement Patterns

Flexion and Extension. Flexion and extension occur at both the atlanto-occipital and the atlanto-axial region. The total flexion and extension between both levels is nearly equal, with a tendency for the articulation between the atlas and occiput to have slightly greater flexion and extension capabilities than that between the atlas and axis.[62] There are about 25 degrees of combined flexion and extension at the occiput-atlas articulation and 20 degrees at the atlas-axis articulation (see Tables 4–5 and 4–6). As noted in the tables, there is a wide variation in the amount of motion purported to be present. Part of the variability in this instance, however, is the difficulty in getting accurate, reproducible measurements between these two highly specialized articulations with even the most sophisticated technology. Caution in interpretation must, therefore, be that much greater in assessments of segmental motion between these levels, using palpation techniques.

Flexion of the occiput on the atlas is limited by the bony contact between the anterior rim of the foramen magnum and the superior surface of the dens (Fig. 4–23). To better visualize this, it is important to remember that the dens functionally serves as the body of the atlas; thus, it is in proximity to abut the rim of the foramen magnum during flexion, especially because no intervertebral disc is present. Extension is limited by the connective tissue restraints of the tectorial and anterior atlanto-occipital membranes.[62] The inherent stability of this region is evidenced by the fact that the amount of sagittal plane translation between the occiput and atlas seldom exceeds 1 mm.[57]

The center of rotation (motion axis) for flexion and extension between C1 and C2 falls in the region of the dens. Restraints to excessive flexion or extension are analyzed using this as the reference point. Additionally, the joint capsules are loose and the articulations are relatively flat to biconvex. Therefore, capsular and bony anatomy

Table 4–5. Occiput-Atlas Range of Motion—Total Flexion and Extension

Panjabi et al[51]	Penning[53]	White & Panjabi[62]
24	30	13

Table 4–6. Atlas-Axis Range of Motion—Total Flexion and Extension

Dvorak et al[15]	Panjabi et al[51]	Penning[63]	White & Panjabi[62]	Poirier & Charpey[62]
12	24	30	13	11

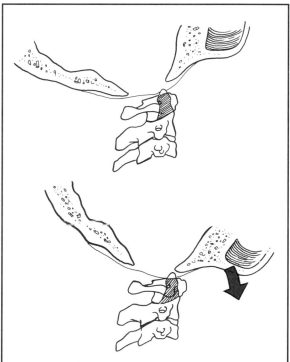

Figure 4–23. The rim of the foramen magnum checks flexion as the occiput impacts on the dens.

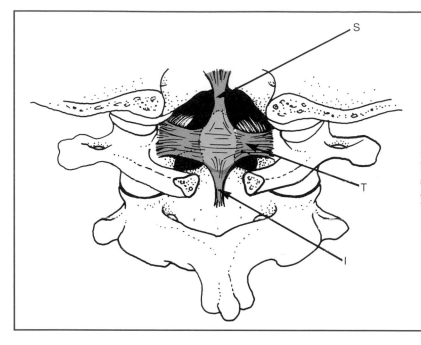

Figure 4–24. Components of the cruciate ligament. I, inferior band of the cruciate ligament; S, superior longitudinal band of the cruciate ligament; T, transverse band of the cruciate ligament.

contribute minimally to stability in the region.[33] The configuration of the dens closely nestled within the anterior arch of the atlas and tightly surrounded by the transverse ligament provides not only the stability, but also the necessary checkreins against excessive flexion and extension movements. Ruptures of the transverse ligament most frequently occur in an older age group (fifth decade) with the mechanism of injury most commonly being a fall resulting in acute flexion of the neck.[38] Clinical symptoms vary, depending on the displacement of the vertebrae. Patients with less significant displacement may experience severe upper neck pain; signifi-

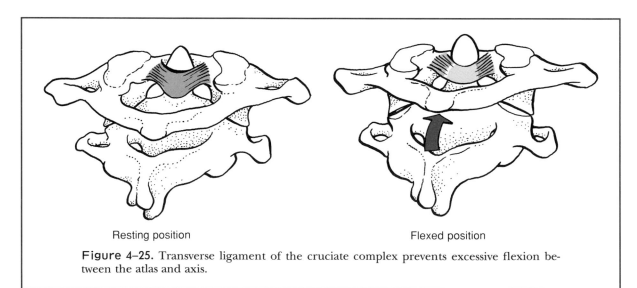

Resting position

Flexed position

Figure 4–25. Transverse ligament of the cruciate complex prevents excessive flexion between the atlas and axis.

Table 4–7. Occiput-Atlas Range of Motion—Rotation in One Direction

White & Panjabi[62]	Penning[53]	Dvorak et al[15]	Panjabi et al[51]	Clark[12]
0	1.0	4.3	3.6	4.8

cant displacement results in neurological deficit that may be a mixed pattern or Brown-Séquard syndrome.[38]

The transverse ligament is a component of the cruciate ligament (see below). The term *cruciate* is used because of the ascending and descending aspects of the ligament, which, when combined with the orientation of the transverse ligament, form a shape like a cross (Fig. 4–24). The transverse ligament is 7 to 8 mm thick, which gives the ligament great strength.[62] During flexion of the atlas on the axis, the dens is pushed posteriorly against the strong transverse ligament, thus limiting further anterior sagittal rotation (Fig. 4–25). In addition, the normal anterior translation that would occur with flexion is effectively checked by the bony and transverse ligament arrangement.

Rotation. A small amount of rotation occurs between the occiput and atlas (Table 4–7). Various sources in the literature place the total amount (sum of right and left rotation) between 1 and 8 degrees.[12, 16, 51] The shape of the bony articulations and the alar ligaments are the major restraints to rotation and prevent excessive rotatory capabilities.

In contrast, the rotatory capability between C1 and C2 far exceed that between the occiput and atlas or between any of the lower cervical segments (Table 4–8). Rotatory range of motion to one side ranges from 34 to 47 degrees, with an average of 40 degrees.[15, 16, 58] Nearly 60 per cent of the total amount of axial rotation available in

the cervical spine is located within the upper two articulations.[62] Mimura and associates suggest that axial rotation between the occiput and C2 vertebral level accounts for 70 per cent of the axial rotation of the entire cervical spine.[44] About 55 per cent of the total rotation of the cervical spine occurs at the atlanto-axial level.[54]

The inferior articular processes of the atlas and the superior articular processes of the axis are relatively flat to convex.[33] The articular surfaces provide the opportunity for a great deal of rotary motion but at the expense of inherent stability. Consider the limitation in atlas-axis rotation if a concave-convex relation was present instead. With the center of rotation for rotary motion located within the region of the dens, a concave-convex relation between the apophyseal joints would curtail the rotary motion. By not having a concave surface, the superior facets of C2 do not provide a bony block to rotation between C1 and C2. Instead, movement of the inferior facet can continue in either an anterior or a posterior direction, which increases range of motion between these two vertebrae.

When viewing lateral radiographs of this region, the shape of the articular facets of C1 and C2 might be difficult to fully appreciate. It should be remembered, however, that the articular cartilage forms the flattened or convex surfaces, rather than the bony elements themselves.[62]

As a result of this arrangement, the rotary motion of C1 on C2 is also coupled to a vertical translation of the same two vertebrae (Fig. 4–26). A simple way to think of this coupling is to visualize that as the head is turned in one direction (C1 is rotating on C2, for example), the inferior facets of C1 "descend" the convex superior facets of C2, in effect making the cervical spine relatively "shorter." Returning the head to the forward position requires the inferior facets to "reclimb" the convexity of the superior facets, in effect making the person "taller" because of the vertical translation. This subtle motion allows the statement to be made that rotation and vertical translation are coupled at the C1-2 articulation.

Translation between the occiput and atlas is insignificant and impossible to assess without sophisticated radiographic analysis. Likewise, the amount of translation between C1 and C2 is only 2 to 3 mm.[27] Again, sophisticated radiographic techniques are required to assess this.

Table 4–8. Atlas-Axis Range of Motion—Rotation in One Direction

Panjabi et al[51]	Dvorak et al[15]	Penning[53]	White & Panjabi[62]	Werne[58]
39	41	40	47	47

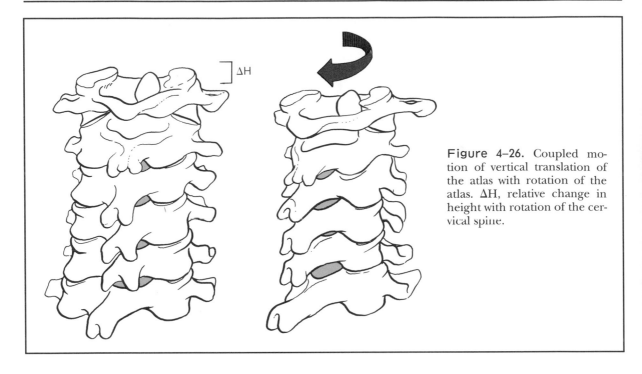

Figure 4–26. Coupled motion of vertical translation of the atlas with rotation of the atlas. ΔH, relative change in height with rotation of the cervical spine.

LIGAMENTS OF THE CERVICAL SPINE

Although some of the ligaments have been referred to above, it is useful to group the ligaments separate from the discussion of bony anatomy to better visualize their relations and functions.

Ligamentum Nuchae and Supraspinous Ligament

The supraspinous ligaments have, for the most part, evolved into the large, thick ligamentum nuchae in the cervical spine.[20, 31] The ligamentum nuchae extends from the C7 or T1 spinous processes to the external occipital protuberance. It is an extremely important supporting structure for the head and neck in quadrupeds. Gravitational forces place a flexion moment on the head and neck of the quadruped that is resisted by the strong ligamentum nuchae. In the human, there is also a flexion moment on the head and neck because of the anterior location of the center of

mass of the head. One of the structures responsible for countering this flexion moment is the ligamentum nuchae.

The deeper fibers of the supraspinous ligament merge and reinforce the interspinous ligaments. In the cervical spine, the interspinous ligaments are not as well developed as in other areas of the spine.

Ligamentum Flavum and Posterior Atlanto-Occipital and Atlantoaxial Membranes

The ligamentum flavum is an important ligament in the cervical spine. By attaching to the anterior portion of the vertebral arch and extending inferiorly to the superior border of the lamina of the vertebra below, it is in a position to serve as one of the posterior boundaries of the spinal canal (Fig. 4–27).

During flexion of the cervical spine, the ligamentum flavum is stretched; when the spine is extended, the tensile force is removed from the ligament. The ligamentum flavum must decrease in length by about 40 per cent in moving from

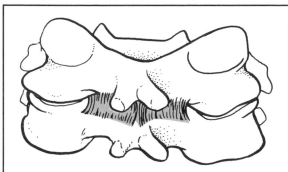

Figure 4–27. Ligamentum flavum, which bridges the space between adjacent lamina.

flexion to extension.[53] Extension does not typically result in the ligamentum flavum buckling into the spinal canal and impinging on the spinal cord because of the high proportion of elastic fibers compared with other ligaments. This high proportion of elastic fibers assures that despite such a decrease in length, the spinal cord does not become impinged because the decrease in length needed for the extension motion is accommodated by the elasticity of the ligament rather than by buckling. During extension, the ligamentum flavum retracts and thickens by redistributing its volume and relaxing its state of pretension.[55] Loss of disc height has the potential to result in infolding of the ligamentum flavum, as do age-related changes caused by degeneration. Buckling of the ligamentum flavum during cervical extension may then occur and contribute to spinal canal stenosis.

The ligamentum flavum also contributes to the formation of the anterior wall of the apophyseal joint capsule. Therefore, the structures affected with marked degenerative changes of the apophyseal joint include not only the articular cartilage, bone, and posterior apophyseal joint capsule, but also the ligamentum flavum. A hypertrophic ligamentum flavum alters the space and anatomical relations of two vital areas: the spinal canal and the intervertebral foramen.

The ligamentum flavum is present between the laminae of C2 and C3 and all the vertebral segments caudal to this level. Above the C2 level, the ligamentum flavum is replaced by the posterior atlantoaxial and atlanto-occipital membranes, which course superiorly to attach to the foramen magnum from their inferior attachments to the posterior rings of the axis and atlas. The structure of the posterior atlanto-occipital and atlantoaxial membranes results in different mechanical considerations when compared with the structure of the ligamentum flavum seen at lower cervical levels. Although having a high proportion of elastic fibers, the ligamentum flavum is thick and strong, which gives it a stiffness important for cervical stability.

The absence of the ligamentum flavum at the segmental level where most rotary motion occurs (C1 and C2) is noteworthy. If the ligamentum flavum were present, the amount of axial rotation capable between these two segments would be markedly lessened. Instead, the ligamentum flavum is replaced with the broad and lax posterior atlantoaxial membrane, which permits a much wider range of motion between C1 and C2.

Apophyseal Joint Capsular Ligaments

The capsules of the apophyseal joints are referred to as capsular ligaments. As in most areas of the spine, the orientation of the capsule fibers are 90 degrees to the plane of the facets. They traverse nearly a 180-degree arc as they course around the articular processes, starting at the transverse process and continuing around to the lamina. The total length of the capsular ligaments is 5 to 7 mm.[31] Although they are thick and dense, laxity of the joint capsules is necessary to allow for the wide range of cervical motion, including the translation capabilities.

The joint capsules are innervated by the medial branches of the cervical dorsal rami from C2 to C8 (Fig. 4–28).[4] There is experimental evidence that the apophyseal joint capsules can serve as a source of pain.[6] Dwyer and co-workers have demonstrated that the apophyseal joints can be responsible for referred pain patterns as well.[18] Using injections into the cervical apophyseal joint space as experimental stimulus, they found that 1 mm of contrast fluid was sufficient to cause capsular distention and initiate local and referred pain. The C2-3 pain pattern extended up to the head; the C3-4 pain pattern encompassed the region approximately over the levator scapulae muscle but not extending over the occiput; the C5-6 pattern extended over the superior aspect

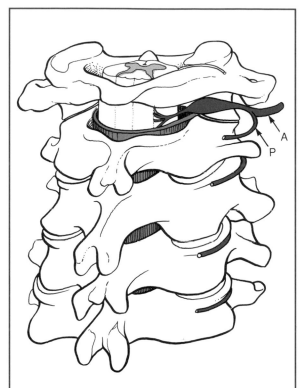

Figure 4–28. Medial branches of the posterior rami innervating the cervical apophyseal joints. A, anterior ramus; P, posterior ramus.

Compressive forces on articular cartilage initially result in fibrillation of the cartilage surface. As the degenerative process advances, these fibrillations gradually become wider clefts and, ultimately, expose the subchondral bone. Shear forces exert a different type of degenerative change, as evidenced by the cartilage changes that occur in the facets of the lumbar spine.[45] The articular cartilage subjected to shear forces begins to split parallel to the cartilage-bone interface and remains continuous with the articular capsule. The damaged articular cartilage with its attachment to the capsule resembles a meniscus and may be vulnerable to becoming lodged within the joint, perhaps resulting in the locking phenomena often described by patients. The block to the joint might be the template of articular cartilage that remains attached to the periphery of the joint capsule.[45] Whether this is a similar phenomena in the cervical spine remains to be investigated, but it is suggested here for consideration of the significance of shear forces across the apophyseal joints.

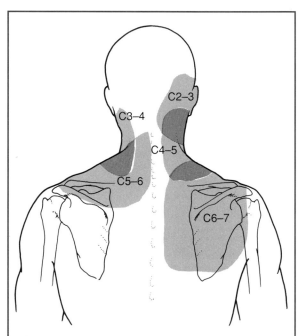

Figure 4–29. Referred pain patterns suggested with pathology of the apophyseal joints. (Adapted from Dwyer A, April C, Bogduk N: Cervical zygapophyseal joint pain patterns. Spine 15:453–457, 1990.)

of the scapula above the level of the scapular spine; and the C6-7 level extended inferiorly toward the inferior angle of the scapula (Fig. 4–29).[18] This study suggests that headaches over the posterior occipital region might be a result of referred pain from the C2-3 apophyseal joints. As in the lumbar spine, there is strong suggestion that the referred pain pattern of the apophyseal joint occurs in a pattern characteristic with the segmental origin of the somatic tissues.

A second theoretical source of pain from the apophyseal joints is the degeneration of the articular cartilage of the facets, which ultimately increases the weight-bearing requirements of the subchondral bone or perhaps results in a mechanical or chemical synovitis that affects the joint capsule. The articular cartilage of the cervical facets is subject to both compression and shear forces, which typically occur simultaneously during movement.

Anterior Longitudinal Ligament and Anterior Atlanto-Occipital Membrane

The anterior longitudinal ligament is thin and translucent in the cervical spine, which is opposite the arrangement in the lumbar spine.[31] It is attached to the vertebral bodies and the intervertebral discs at the level of the third cervical vertebra and all the caudal segments. The ligament extends superiorly to attach to the body of the axis and then continues superiorly to the body of the atlas. It continues upward to the occiput, where it is referred to as the anterior atlanto-occipital membrane.

Posterior Longitudinal Ligament and Tectorial Membrane

The posterior longitudinal ligament is widest in the cervical region and narrows as it approaches the lumbar region. The width and thickness of the posterior longitudinal ligament in the cervical region allow it to serve as an excellent barrier against posterior protrusion of inter-vertebral disc material. This feature offers protection to the spinal cord. The posterior longitudinal ligament also limits flexion and intervertebral distraction.[60] Whereas the anterior atlanto-occipital membrane is the continuation of the anterior longitudinal ligament on the anterior aspect of the vertebral body of the atlas, the tectorial membrane is the continuation of the posterior longitudinal ligament in the upper two segments of the cervical spine. The tectorial membrane is a broad, strong membrane that covers the dens and its associated cruciate ligament as it courses superiorly to attach to the anterior rim of the foramen magnum and blend with the cranial dura mater (Fig. 4–30).[65]

Ligaments Related to the Upper Cervical Spine

The following ligaments of the upper cervical spine do not have comparable counterparts in the lower cervical spine, as has been the case with the previously described ligaments. It has already been mentioned that the occipito-atlanto-axial segment can be considered as a single functional

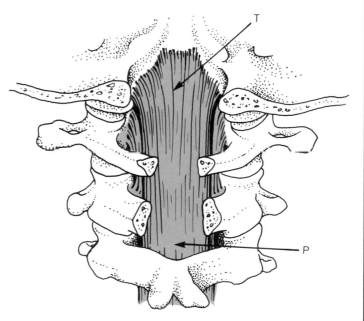

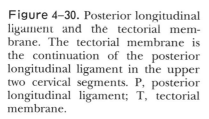

Figure 4–30. Posterior longitudinal ligament and the tectorial membrane. The tectorial membrane is the continuation of the posterior longitudinal ligament in the upper two cervical segments. P, posterior longitudinal ligament; T, tectorial membrane.

unit. This is especially evident when the ligamentous attachments of this complex are analyzed. Ligaments that connect the occiput to the atlas include the articular capsules and the anterior, posterior, and lateral atlanto-occipital membranes. A second group of ligaments connect the occiput to the axis and include the cruciate ligament complex, tectorial membrane, alar ligaments, and apical dental ligament.[19, 21] It has been demonstrated experimentally that the most important of the two groups in regard to stability is the latter.[58]

Although the upper cervical spine complex often is divided into two distinct components—the occipito-atlanto and atlanto-axial articulations—both are functionally interwoven by this ligamentous complex in such a way that the essential movement of the upper cervical spine actually takes place between the occiput and the axis, with the atlas serving as a bearing to help regulate this motion.[53] Although the theoretical effects of various mobilization maneuvers of the occiput on the atlas are implied, such discussion leads only toward a more thorough understanding of the joint arthrokinematics of this segment. They serve little practical value because the occiput does not move independently on the atlas. When the attachments of the alar ligaments are appreciated, it is immediately apparent that any occipital motion also directly affects the motion of the axis (Fig. 4–31). Put more succinctly, any

occipital motion immediately and directly results in specific forces being imparted to the axis. The paired alar ligaments and the apical ligament connect the axis with the occipital bone and assure that this is the case.

Cruciate Ligament Complex

The cruciate ligament complex is an important stabilizer of the occiput-atlas-axis region (see Fig. 4–24). This ligamentous complex sits immediately anterior to the tectorial membrane. The most significant portion of the cruciate ligament is the transverse ligament, which attaches on either side of the atlas and courses posterior to the dens. The complete ligament complex is referred to as the cruciate ligament because an ascending band and a descending band arise from the transverse ligament, forming a structure shaped like a cross. The superior band courses cranially and attaches to the margin of the foramen magnum, and the descending band is attached caudally to the body of C2. In general, the transverse band is twice as thick as the ascending or descending band. The transverse ligament is the primary stabilizer, preventing anterior translation of C1 on C2. Excessive anterior translation between these two segments results in the dens being compressed against the ventral surface of the spinal cord.

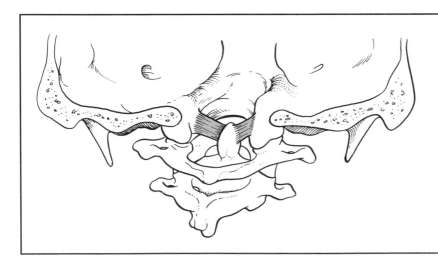

Figure 4–31. The alar ligaments serve to make the occiput, atlas, and axis move as one functional unit.

Because the transverse ligament is located posterior to the axis of upper cervical motion, the ligament prevents flexion of the occiput-atlas complex on the axis.[59] During flexion, the atlas tilts forward and translates anteriorly. This motion is strongly resisted because the transverse ligament is brought directly against the posterior aspect of the dens.

Alar Ligaments

The alar and apical ligaments are located immediately anterior to the cruciate ligament complex. Thus, from superficial to deep (posterior to anterior), the ligaments of the upper cervical spine are the tectorial membrane, cruciate ligament, and alar and apical ligaments. The alar ligaments consist of two portions: one attaches to the atlas (atlantoalar) and the other attaches to the occiput (occipitoalar; see Fig. 4–31).[16, 17] These ligaments are short and often blended with the capsules of the occipitoatlanto joints and the atlantodental joint. The ligaments appear as strong rounded cords on either side of the upper part of the dens.

Each alar ligament relaxes on extension of the head but tautens with flexion. The alar ligaments are one of the main restraints to occipital flexion. They also form the main restraint to excessive axial rotation between the occiput and atlas and the atlas and axis.[17] Rotation to the right is limited by the left alar ligament and rotation to the left is prevented by the right alar ligament, although, depending on the size and specific bony attachments, both ligaments can simultaneously limit rotation, especially with varying degrees of flexion.

These ligaments are strong when subjected to experimental tests of rotational strain.[17] It is unlikely that they rupture with rotational forces alone. It would be more common to have bone avulsions or fractures of the dens instead of ligamentous rupture.[23] Even though their checkrein functions are impressive, their attachments clearly emphasize the functional relation that results between the occiput and C2.

Apical Ligaments

The apical ligaments are attached to the tip of the dens and extend superiorly to attach to the anterior rim of the foramen magnum. These small ligaments are bordered by the two alar ligaments.

Biomechanical Considerations of Stretching

It is important to consider the effects of various stretching maneuvers on the cervical spine because one of the purported effects is to alter the state of the connective tissue elements of the cervical spine. Ligamentous strength is dependent on the collagen fiber and ground substance composition as well as the cross-sectional area. When the major ligamentous and capsular checkreins to movement in the cervical spine are analyzed, it is apparent that many different ligamentous structures must be considered to limit movement and contribute to the overall stability of the cervical spine.

For example, most of the posterior ligamentous structures, such as the ligamentum nuchae, capsular ligaments, and ligamentum flavum, tauten with flexion because they are located posterior to the center of rotation for cervical flexion and extension. In addition, the same flexion maneuver increases tensile stresses in the fascia surrounding the musculature and in the posterior aspect of the annulus fibrosus. The annulus fibrosus offers a significant restraint to the flexion force because the anterior aspect resists the compressive stress that occurs with flexion and the posterior annulus strongly resists tensile and shear stresses.

From a biomechanical standpoint, it appears difficult to produce permanent deformation of the connective tissue with the typical stretching maneuvers applied in the clinical situation. Taking any of the above-named connective tissue structures into the plastic range of their viscoelastic capacity does not appear reasonable. In addition, the clinician would want to question why such an effect would be indicated because permanently elongating tissue by taking it to its plastic range would leave it less able to withstand subsequent tensile stresses placed on it.

The micro and macro traumas that the connective tissue is subjected to often results in loss of normal range of motion because of degenerative changes. These weakened inert tissues can be altered with manual and mechanical techniques because they are not as resilient as uninjured tissue. It is important that as much motion as possible be restored to minimize the catabolic changes and further weakening of tissues that occur with inactivity.

The various stretching, traction, mobilization, and manipulation maneuvers probably have a more direct effect on the neuromuscular apparatus, which results in immediate changes in range of motion. Perhaps it is the set of the muscles, with their intimate relations to many of the capsular, ligamentous, and fascial structures, that allows for frequently seen changes in range of motion and movement patterns with the application of such treatment techniques.

Intervertebral Disc

In the cervical spine, an intervertebral disc is present between each vertebra except between the occiput and atlas and the atlas and axis. This arrangement further demonstrates the uniqueness of the occiput-atlas-axis articulations when compared with the remainder of the cervical spine. In many aspects, the disc of the cervical spine is typical of that of other regions of the spine, but there some features are unique. The intervertebral discs form joints in the axial skeleton that are responsible for conferring flexibility to the spine.[29] In both the cervical and the lumbar spine, the intervertebral disc has an elliptical shape. The liability of such a shape is that it leads to posterior and posterolateral stress concentrations as a result of torsion. The advantage, however, is that such an arrangement places a large proportion of the reinforcing annular fibers posterior to the axis of forward bending. Complete failure of the posterior annulus is thus potentially avoided.[29]

The intervertebral disc consists of the gelatinous nucleus pulposus surrounded peripherally by the fibrocartilaginous annulus fibrosus and superiorly and inferiorly by the cartilaginous end plates (Fig. 4–32). It is important to recognize the cartilaginous end plate as a component of the intervertebral disc because the collagen fibers are continuous between the annulus fibrosus and the cartilage of the end plate. The nucleus pulposus is essentially encapsulated by the collagen framework of the annulus fibrosus and cartilaginous end plates.[7] The boundary between the inner annulus fibrosus and the outer nucleus pulposus is not clearly defined.

The cervical discs are different from the thoracic and lumbar discs in that they do not extend to the lateral rims of the vertebral bodies. In this lateral area is located the uncinate processes, which extend upward from the subjacent vertebral body to make contact with the lateral margins of the vertebra above the disc.

The annulus fibrosus consists of crimped collagen fibrils organized into concentric lamellae. The fiber directions alternate by about 90 degrees with each successive layer. The fiber orientation usually is between 30 and 40 degrees to the horizontal. The proportion of collagen increases from the inner to the outer annulus fibrosus.[29] The strength and oblique orientation of the annular fibers, combined with their extremely strong attachment to the peripheral regions of the vertebral body, result in the annulus fibrosus being the primary checkrein for any horizontal translation between adjacent vertebrae.

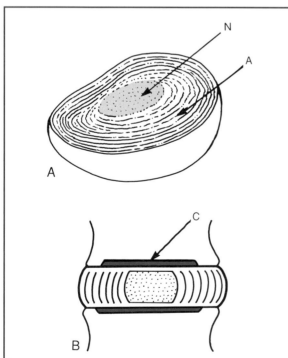

Figure 4–32. Components of the intervertebral disc. The cartilaginous end plates are also considered a component of the intervertebral disc. A, concentric rings of the annulus fibrosus; C, cartilaginous end plate; N, region of the nucleus pulposus.

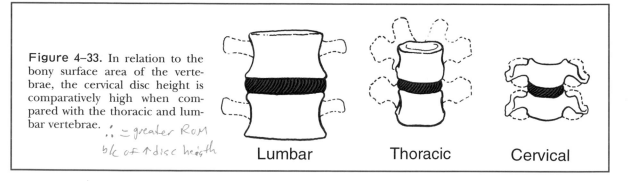

Figure 4–33. In relation to the bony surface area of the vertebrae, the cervical disc height is comparatively high when compared with the thoracic and lumbar vertebrae. ∴ = greater ROM b/c of ↑disc height

Lumbar   **Thoracic**   **Cervical**

The nucleus pulposus consists of a hydrated gel of proteoglycans with some collagen.[29] Because of this macromolecular makeup, water accounts for more than 80 per cent of the weight of the nucleus. Negatively charged sulfate groups are readily available in the macromolecules to attract and bind water. Collagen, by comparison, accounts for only 5 per cent of the weight of the nucleus.[29] In relation to its surface area, the cervical disc height is comparatively high, which in part is one of the major reasons for the large amount of motion present in the cervical spine (Fig. 4–33). In addition, the cervical discs are wedge-shaped, being of greater height anteriorly than posteriorly, and therefore, they are the primary reason for the configuration of the cervical lordosis.[36]

The intervertebral discs play an important role in distributing pressure over the vertebral body surface during various bending maneuvers (Fig. 4–34). Without intervertebral discs, bending

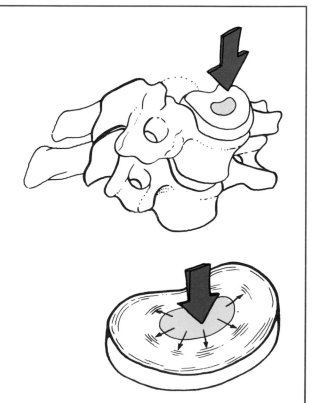

Figure 4–34. Distribution of pressure by the nucleus pulposus against the walls of the annulus fibrosus. The compressive forces are redirected in a tangential manner against the inner walls of the annulus fibrosus.

would cause a concentration of compression eccentrically over a small focal area of the vertebrae.[2] With the deformable intervertebral disc interposed between the vertebral bodies, the same force is distributed over a much larger bony surface, which helps to distribute compressive forces over a larger area.

Although several studies regarding lumbar intradiscal pressure are available, few studies have been done on intradiscal pressure of the cervical discs. The cervical intervertebral disc can be assumed to exert a swelling pressure because of the proteoglycan matrix of the nucleus, which attracts water. Because the nucleus contains a greater proportion of proteoglycans than the annulus, the nucleus attracts more water by osmosis and causes the extracellular matrix to exert a swelling pressure against the annulus and cartilaginous end plates.[29]

Hattori and colleagues studied intradiscal pressure in the cervical spine in vivo.[24] With the patient in a supine position, a needle-type semiconductor pressure transducer was placed into the C4-5, C5-6, and C6-7 intervertebral discs under fluoroscopic control, and the patient was brought to the sitting position. Both normal and degenerated discs were evaluated for pressure changes seen with various movements. In normal discs, the highest pressures occurred when the neck was taken into extension; flexion produced the next highest pressures. Rotation and lateral bending, which are strongly coupled motions, had the least increase in intradiscal pressure. Their methods fail to note whether the motion was active or passive, which does not allow for a hypothesis to be drawn regarding the change in intervertebral pressure caused by the compressive force of muscle contraction.

In Hattori's study, the intervertebral disc pressures measured in the sitting position were 1.4 times greater than those measured in the supine position.[24] Cervical traction applied with a head halter resulted in a decrease in intradiscal pressure proportional to the traction force. With a 10-kg weight, the pressure decreased by 57 per cent with traction forces applied in the supine position and by 44 per cent with traction forces applied in the sitting position. The authors concluded that it might be reasonable to assume about a 50 per cent decrease in intradiscal pressure with a 10-kg traction force.

Hattori and co-workers also noted that degenerated discs present a slightly different and highly unpredictable picture.[24] With increasing disc degeneration, there is less intradiscal pressure. Some intervertebral discs exhibited higher pressures in extension, whereas others showed higher pressures in flexion. The pressure decreased with cervical traction, and with the 10-kg traction force, the pressure often went to zero. More studies are needed to assess the changes in intradiscal pressure that occur as a result of postural position and muscle contraction.

Disc pressure exerted by the hydrated nucleus pulposus is an important mechanical feature of the intervertebral disc. Collagen fibers can reinforce a tissue only if they are oriented so that they can be stretched by an applied force.[29] The radial component of the pressure exerted by the nucleus pulposus increases tension on the annular fibers so that they become stretched. When such a force is applied to the annulus, the collagen fibers are able to resist buckling (see Fig. 4–34).

Much of the annulus fibrosus of the cervical spine discs has been shown to be innervated.[8] The primary source of these nerve fibers is the ventral rami, from which the sinuvertebral and vertebral nerves branch. Nerve fibers enter the disc from the posterolateral direction and course both parallel and perpendicular to the collagen bundles of the annulus fibrosus. Nerve fibers are seen throughout the disc but are most numerous in the middle third.[43] These nerve fibers are free nerve endings and resemble pacinian corpuscles. Therefore, the nerve fibers may subserve a mechanoreceptor function as well as a nociceptive function.

It is important to recognize the implication for the pain resulting from provocation discography as well as discogenic pain. Provocation discography is the injection of contrast medium or normal saline solution that results in distention of the annulus fibrosus which causes the afferent nerves of the annulus to discharge.[8, 34] Alternatively, disc degradation might result in the intervertebral disc being a primary source of pain because of the chemical stimulation of the nociceptors located within the innervated portions of the disc.

Disc Degeneration

Pathophysiological changes of the intervertebral disc are probably a combination of biomechanical and biochemical factors. Morphological changes occur that result in various pathological states, such as herniations of the nucleus pulposus through the cartilaginous end plate (Schmorl's nodes), fissuring and cracking of the annulus fibrosus, diffuse bulging or focal extrusion of the disc material that can be composed of various quantities of nucleus pulposus and cartilaginous end plate material, thinning of the disc that results in increased approximation between the articular facets, and altered kinematics of the intervertebral foramen.

Disc degeneration appears to occur naturally with age. Most cervical spines show evidence of degeneration after the fourth decade, with even greater degenerative evidence present after the fifth decade.[2] Disc degeneration most frequently is noticed at the C5-6 and C6-7 levels.[14]

With degeneration, the ability of the intervertebral disc to imbibe water, and thus provide for load distribution, declines. This is due to the loss of the negatively charged proteoglycans, which bind water. Because of this loss, the osmotic swelling pressure within the intervertebral disc decreases. Because the nucleus pulposus has a greater proportion of proteoglycans than collagen, this change in water-imbibing capabilities affects the nucleus more than the annulus. The same loss of proteoglycans in the annulus has an overall effect on its mechanical properties, however. It is thought that the loss of proteoglycans in the annulus increases the likelihood of failure of overstressed regions of the annulus.[26] These changes alter the mechanics of the intervertebral disc, especially loss of the ability of the nucleus to convert a vertical load into a tangential force against the walls of the annulus.

Although the mechanical pressure of a bulging disc against structures within the spinal canal can be a sequelae of disc degeneration, it has become increasingly evident that concurrent biochemical changes must also be present for the symptoms and signs of pain and functional changes to occur. Previously avascular nuclear material has now come into contact with the bloodstream and can initiate an autoimmune response.[49] Nuclear material that continues to leak through defects in the annulus fibrosus appears to be able to potentiate the inflammatory process.[42] The avascularity of the intervertebral disc, which isolates it from the immune system, predisposes it to in-

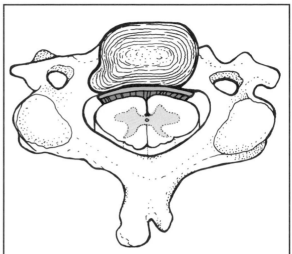

Figure 4–35. Cervical disc protrusions usually occur laterally because of the width of the posterior longitudinal ligament.

tense inflammatory reactions when sequestration occurs.[49]

The location of the intervertebral disc protrusion in the spinal canal accounts in part for the signs and symptoms seen in the patient. Because of the width of the posterior longitudinal ligament, intraforaminal herniations are more frequent than midline herniations (Fig. 4–35).[2] Pressure on the nerve roots may render them ischemic. In addition, a nerve root coursing over a disc bulge is placed under a greater degree of tension (Fig. 4–36). This tension may induce local inflammatory changes with a long-range sequela of fibrosis around the nerve root. Most cervical radiculopathies are localized to the C5-6 or C6-7 level.[25]

In addition to causing radiculopathies, cervical intervertebral disc protrusions may result in myelopathy because the spinal cord occupies most of the cervical spinal canal. As a result, upper motor neuron signs might be present with cervical disc lesions.[9] Patients with developmental cervical stenosis are predisposed to cervical myelopathy and, therefore, have even less ability to accommodate cervical disc protrusions. The reduction in the volume of the spinal canal causing cervical myelopathy can be any combination of intervertebral disc bulges, hypertrophic ligamentum flavum, foraminal osteophytes, and hypertro-

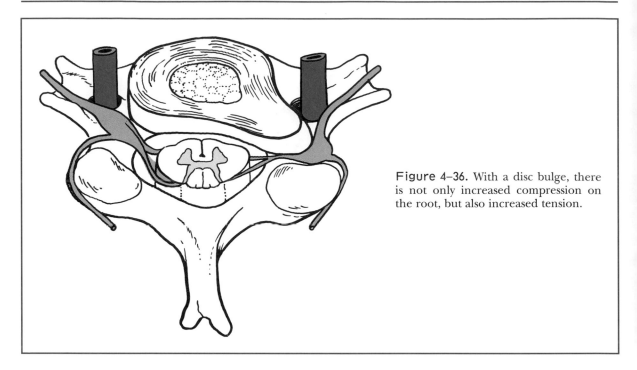

Figure 4–36. With a disc bulge, there is not only increased compression on the root, but also increased tension.

phy of the lamina or facets, for example. Note also how flexion of the cervical spine can result in the spinal cord being stretched over a significant disc bulge or vertebral body osteophyte, which can result in a dynamic cervical spine stenosis (Fig. 4–37).[10]

CERVICAL SPONDYLOSIS

The previous discussion regarding intervertebral disc degeneration provides the basis for understanding the clinical importance of cervical spondylosis. A review of the syndrome of cervical

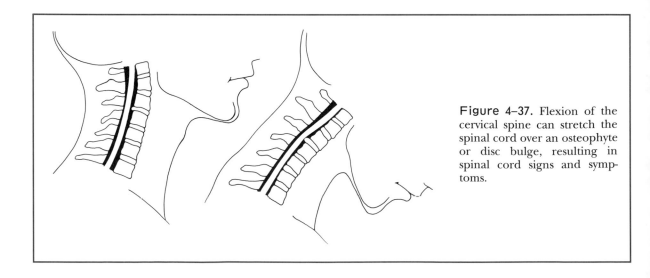

Figure 4–37. Flexion of the cervical spine can stretch the spinal cord over an osteophyte or disc bulge, resulting in spinal cord signs and symptoms.

spondylosis allows the functional anatomy related to the articulations to be considered in a more complete manner.

Cervical spondylosis is essentially a degenerative disease of the cervical spine, with the process initiated by changes in the intervertebral disc. The clinical relevance is that the degenerative process results in compressive or tensile forces to the neural structures, resulting in radiculopathy, myelopathy, or claudication phenomena. Primary neck pain with no radicular or myelopathical involvement is also a potential sequela. Cervical spondylosis that results in myelopathy is the most serious consequence of intervertebral disc degeneration. Such a spondylitic myelopathy is the most common cervical cord disorder during and after middle age.[13, 39]

The size of the spinal canal is of great importance in considering the resultant effects of cervical spondylosis. Compromise of the canal can occur for a multitude of reasons, but for the purposes of this chapter, only those structures that have been previously discussed are mentioned. The spinal canal has the potential to be compromised through protrusion or extrusion of disc material, subluxation of the vertebrae, folding of the ligamentum flavum, or development of bony osteophytes in the region of the vertebral bodies, uncinate processes, or neural arch.[11] The compressive phenomenon affects not only the nervous tissue directly, but also, perhaps more importantly, the blood vessels that supply the spinal cord. Radiculopathy caused by cervical spondylosis may also be the result of disc protrusion or osteophytes that develop on the uncinate processes or apophyseal joints. Signs and symptoms related to myelopathy and radiculopathy are discussed in Chapter 2. The purpose of mentioning these clinical conditions at this point is to underscore the intricate relation between the various articulations of the cervical spine and the neural and vascular framework.

Conversely, degenerative disease of the cervical spine frequently occurs in the absence of clinical symptoms. Boden and associates have demonstrated that magnetic imaging scans of subjects with no history of symptoms indicative of cervical disease were interpreted as demonstrating an abnormality in 19 per cent of the subjects.[2] Furthermore, these false-positive diagnoses occurred in 14 per cent of the subjects younger than age 40 and in 28 per cent of those older than 40. The most frequently diagnosed abnormalities were herniated nucleus pulposus and foraminal stenosis. It is essential, then, that abnormalities seen with imaging studies be clearly matched with clinical signs and symptoms.

SUMMARY

To detail the articulations of the cervical spine in a comprehensive manner, it is necessary to divide the spine into lower and upper segments. Structures unique to the cervical spine, including the uncinate processes, housing for the intervertebral discs, structure of the transverse processes, and biomechanics unique to the cervical spine are discussed in this chapter. In addition, the ligaments of the upper cervical spine are presented to appreciate that the occiput-atlas-axis segments are more locally considered as one functional unit rather than as three independent elements.

The articulations and their various support components represent important aspects of the specialized connective tissue system referred to in Chapter 1: bones, articular cartilage, intervertebral discs, and support ligaments. These tissues are continually stressed by the forces of gravity and movement.

Chapters 5 and 6 develop the assessment and treatment technique considerations for the cervical spine. A clear understanding of the anatomy and mechanics affords the reader the opportunity to logically apply these techniques, especially as they relate to the diagnosis of activity-related or mechanical neck pain, and treatment objectives, such as biomechanical counseling and the application of controlled forces into the cervical spine, to enhance and promote movement by the patient.

REFERENCES

1. April C, Dwyer A, Bogduk N: Cervical zygapophyseal joint pain patterns. II. A clinical evaluation. Spine 15:458–461, 1990.
2. Boden SD, McCowin PR, Davis DO, et al: Abnormal magnetic resonance scans of the cervical spine in asymptomatic subjects. J Bone Joint Surg [Am] 72:1178–1184, 1990.

3. Boden SD, Wiesel SW, Laws ER, Rothman RH: The Aging Spine. Philadelphia, WB Saunders, 1991.
4. Bogduk N: The clinical anatomy of the cervical dorsal rami. Spine 7:319–330, 1982.
5. Bogduk N, Marsland A: On the concept of the third occipital headache. J Neurol Neurosurg Psychiatry 49:775–780, 1986.
6. Bogduk N, Marsland A: The cervical apophyseal joints as a source of pain. Spine 13:610–617, 1988.
7. Bogduk N, Twomey LT: Clinical Anatomy of the Lumbar Spine. New York, Churchill Livingstone, 1987.
8. Bogduk N, Windsor M, Inglis A: The innervation of the cervical intervertebral discs. Spine 13:2–8, 1988.
9. Bohlmann HH, Emery SE: The pathophysiology of cervical spondylosis and myelopathy. Spine 13:843, 1988.
10. Breig A, Turnbull I, Hassler O: Effects of mechanical stresses on the spinal cord in cervical spondylosis. J Neurosurg 25:45, 1966.
11. Clark CR: Degenerative conditions of the spine. In Frymoyer J (ed): The Adult Spine. New York, Raven Press, 1991, pp 1145–1165.
12. Clark CR, Goel VK, Galles K, Liu YK: Kinematics of the occipito-atlanto-axial complex. Trans Cervical Spine Res Soc 1986.
13. Crandall PH, Gregorius FK: Long-term follow-up of surgical treatment of cervical spondylitic myelopathy. Spine 2:139–146, 1977.
14. DePalma AF, Rothman RH: The Intervertebral Disc. Philadelphia, WB Saunders, 1970, pp 37–38.
15. Dvorak J, Hayek, J, Zehnder R: CT-functional diagnostics of the rotatory instability of the upper cervical spine. II. An evaluation on healthy adults and patients with suspected instability. Spine 12:726, 1987.
16. Dvorak J, Panjabi MM, Gerber M: CT-functional diagnostics of the rotary instability of the upper cervical spine and experimental study in cadavers. Spine 12:197, 1987.
17. Dvorak J, Schneider E, Saldinger P, Rahn B: Biomechanics of the craniocervical region: The alar and transverse ligaments. J Orthop Res 6:452, 1988.
18. Dwyer A, April C, Bogduk N: Cervical zygapophyseal joint pain patterns. I. A study of normal volunteers. Spine 15:453–457, 1990.
19. Evarts CM: Traumatic occipito-atlantal dislocation. A report of a case with survival. J Bone Joint Surg [Am] 52:1653–1660, 1970.
20. Fielding JW, Burstein AA, Frankel VH: The nuchal ligament. Spine 1:3, 1976.
21. Gabriel KR, Mason DE, Carango P: Occipito-atlantal translation in Down's syndrome. Spine 15:997–1002, 1990.
22. Gershon-Cohen J, Budin E, Glauser F: Whiplash fractures of cervicodorsal spinous processes; resemblance to shoveler's fracture. JAMA 155:560, 1954.
23. Goel VK, Winterbottom JM, Schulte KR, et al: Ligamentous laxity across C0-C1-C2 complex. Spine 15:990–996, 1990.
24. Hattori S, Oda H, Kawai S: Cervical intradiscal pressure in movements and traction of the cervical spine. Z Orthop 119:568, 1981.
25. Henderson CM, Hennessy R, Shuey H, et al: Posterior-lateral foraminotomy as an exclusive operative technique for cervical radiculopathy: A review of 846 consecutively operated cases. J Neurosurg 13:504, 1983.
26. Hickey DS, Hukins DWL: Aging changes in the macromolecular organization of the intervertebral disc. An X-ray diffraction and electron microscope study. Spine 7:234–242, 1982.
27. Hohl M, Baker HR: The atlanto-axial joint. J Bone Joint Surg [Am] 46:1739, 1964.
28. Hollinshead WH: Anatomy for Surgeons. Vol. 3. The Back and the Limbs. 2nd ed. New York, Harper & Row, 1969, pp 79–206.
29. Hukins DWL: Disc structure and function. In Ghosh P (ed): The Biology of the Intervertebral Disc. Boca Raton, FL, CRC Press, 1988, pp 1–39.
30. Jeffreys E: Disorders of the Cervical spine. London, Butterworths, 1980, pp 1–147.
31. Johnson RM, Crelin ES, White AA, et al: Some new observations on the functional anatomy of the lower cervical spine. Clin Orthop 111:192, 1975.
32. Jones MD: Cineradiographic studies of the normal cervical spine. Calif Med 93:293, 1960.
33. Kapandji IA: The Physiology of the Joints. Vol. 3. Edinburgh, Churchill Livingstone, 1974.
34. Kikuchi S, MacNab I, Moreau P: Localization of the level of symptomatic cervical disc degeneration. J Bone Joint Surg [Br] 63:272–277, 1981.
35. Krag MH: Biomechanics of the cervical spine. In Frymoyer JW (ed): The Adult Human Spine. New York, Raven Press, 1991, pp 929–965.
36. Lestini WF, Wiesel SW: The pathogenesis of cervical spondylosis. Clin Orthop 239:69–93, 1988.
37. Levine AM, Edwards CC: Treatment of injuries in the C1-C2 complex. Orthop Clin North Am 17:31, 1966.
38. Levine AM, Edwards CC: Traumatic lesions of the occipitoatlantoaxial complex. Clin Orthop 239:53–68, 1989.
39. Lundsford LD, Bissonette DJ, Zorub DS: Anterior surgery for cervical disc disease. II. Treatment of cervical spondylotic myelopathy in 32 cases. J Neurosurg 53:12–19, 1980.
40. Lysell E: Motion in the cervical spine. Acta Orthop Scand Suppl 123:1, 1969.
41. McCall IW, Park WM, O'Brien JP: Induced pain referral from posterior lumbar elements in normal subjects. Spine 4:441–446, 1979.
42. McCarron RF, Wimpee MW, Hudkins PG, Laros GS: The inflammatory effect of the nucleus pulposus: A possible element in the pathogenesis of low back pain. Spine 12:760–764, 1987.
43. Mendel T, Wink CS, Zimny M: Neural elements in human cervical intervertebral discs. Spine 17:132–135, 1992.
44. Mimura M, Moriya H, Watanabe T, et al: Three dimensional motion analysis of the cervical spine with special reference to axial rotation. Spine 14:1135–1139, 1989.
45. Mooney V: Facet syndrome. In Weinstein JN, Wiesl SW (eds): The Lumbar Spine. Philadelphia, WB Saunders, 1990, pp 422–441.
46. Mooney V, Robertson J: The facet syndrome. Clin Orthop 115:149–156, 1976.
47. Morizono Y, Sakou T, Kawaida H: Upper cervical involvement in rheumatoid arthritis. Spine 12:721–725, 1987.
48. Moroney SP, Schultz AB, Miller JAA, Andersson GBJ: Load-displacement properties of lower cervical spine motion segments. J Biomech 21:767, 1988.
49. Naylor A: Epidemiology. In Weinstein JN, Wiesel SW

(eds): The Lumbar Spine. Philadelphia, WB Saunders, 1990, pp 1–32.

50. Orofino C, Sherman MS, Schecter D: Luschka's joint—a degenerative phenomenon. J Bone Joint Surg [Am] 42:853–858, 1960.

51. Panjabi M, Dvorak J, Duranceau J, et al: Three-dimensional movements of the upper cervical spine. Spine 13:726, 1988.

52. Panjabi MM, Summers DJ, Pelker RR, et al: Three dimensional load displacement curves of the cervical spine. J Orthop Res 4:152, 1986.

53. Penning L: Normal movements of the cervical spine. Am J Roentgenol 130:317–326, 1978.

54. Penning L, Wilmink JT: Rotation of the cervical spine. Spine 12:732–738, 1987.

55. Rauschning W: Anatomy and pathology of the cervical spine. In Frymoyer J (ed): The Adult Spine. New York, Raven Press, 1991, pp 907–928.

56. Shapiro R, Youngberg AS, Rothman SL: The differential diagnosis of traumatic lesions of the occipito-atlanto-axial segment. Radiol Clin North Am 11:505–526, 1973.

57. Weisel SW, Rothman RH: Occipital atlantal hypermobility. Spine 4:187, 1979.

58. Werne S: Studies in spontaneous atlas dislocation. Acta Orthop Scand Suppl 23:1, 1957.

59. White AA, Johnson RM, Panjabi MM: Biomechanical analysis of clinical stability in the cervical spine. Clin Orthop 10:85, 1985.

60. White AA, Johnson RM, Panjabi MM, Southwick WO: Biomechanical analysis of clinical stability in the cervical spine. Clin Orthop 109:85, 1975.

61. White AA, Panjabi MM: The clinical biomechanics of the occipito-atlanto-axial complex. Orthop Clin North Am 9:867, 1978.

62. White AA, Panjabi MM: Clinical Biomechanics of the Spine. 2nd ed. Philadelphia, JB Lippincott, 1990.

63. White AA, Southwick WO, DePonte RJ, et al: Relief of pain by anterior cervical spine fusion for spondylosis: A report of 65 patients. J Bone Joint Surg [Am] 55:525, 1973.

64. Williams PL, Warwick R: Gray's Anatomy. 36th ed. Philadelphia, WB Saunders, 1980.

65. Williams PL, Warwick R, Dyson M, Bannister LH: Gray's Anatomy. 37th ed. New York, Churchill Livingstone, 1989.

CHAPTER 5

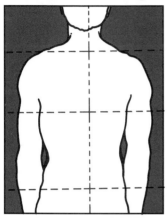

FUNCTIONAL ASSESSMENT OF THE NECK

Disorders related to the cervical spine can present a variety of signs and symptoms because of the many tissues and systems associated with this region. For example, the nervous system is represented by the spinal cord, nerve roots, peripheral nerves, and sympathetic chain; the digestive system, by the pharynx and esophagus; the respiratory system, by the trachea and superior apex of the lung; the skeletal system, by the vertebrae; the vascular system, by such structures as the vertebral artery and subclavian vessels; and the muscular system, by the muscles related to the head, neck, and shoulder girdle. The clinician must be aware of the diversity of potential complaints that the patient may have and the wide spectrum of signs and symptoms that can exist.

The purpose of this chapter is to develop an assessment process that incorporates an understanding of the mechanics of the upper quarter and assesses neural function. A pathomechanical approach to assessment is emphasized because such an approach strives to determine the offending forces that reproduce the familiar symptoms. This forms the basis of the assessment process. The clinician must recognize that unlike the low back, where the various tissues work together to attenuate significant forces and serve as a hub of weight bearing, the neck has intricate neuromus-cular mechanisms that allow for different functions. The cervical spine is distinctly designed to accommodate large ranges of movement and at the same time must counterbalance the weight of the head. The neuromuscular design also allows for an enhanced awareness of movements and a sensory system that is driven by many physical and emotional stressors.

It is a challenge for the clinician to organize the findings of the assessment into a treatment plan that addresses the potential influences on the problem. The assessment process should gather pertinent information from the patient, such as the pain pattern and how the pain pattern results in loss of function. The physical examination focuses on applying forces to the region to determine the stresses, positions, and movements that reproduce familiar pain. Finally, the circumstances (environmental and emotional) that exacerbate the familiar symptoms should be identified.

With the assistance of computed tomography and magnetic resonance imaging, the clinician is able to view the structural pathology of the head and neck. Although the images serve to help measure the spondylitic (degenerative) process, the clinician must make a judgment as to the relation between the changes seen with such radiographic or imaging findings and the results of the assessment.

As the cervical spine begins to demonstrate age-related degenerative changes or changes occur because of progressive overload or as a result of injury, many tissues are simultaneously affected. To strive to precisely identify the one tissue at fault during the assessment process is probably a narrow view of the potential scope of the problem. The painful syndrome often is driven by many factors, all of which must be addressed to maximize the effectiveness of the treatment process.[29]

The assessment process is designed to blend the information gained from the history and the physical examination in such a manner that the pain can be substantiated or reproduced in weight-bearing and non–weight-bearing positions. This yields the pathomechanical diagnosis, which identifies the forces and positions that exacerbate the familiar symptoms. This information should be gained by the application of such forces in the weight-bearing position and then replicated in a recumbent, non–weight-bearing position. The similarities of the response between the weight-bearing and non–weight-bearing positions are then established (matches). The physical parameters that define the similarities form the basis for the treatment process.

DETERMINING THE IRRITABILITY OF THE TISSUE

The clinician must also glean information about the irritability or state of inflammation of the injured tissues from the assessment process. This information is obtained from answers to questions regarding stiffness and soreness during the course of the day and after prolonged postures and from the findings from palpation. An understanding of the inflammatory state can be obtained by asking, "Are you stiffer and sorer in the morning or in the evening?" The patient who describes morning as the worst time of day is informing the clinician of the inflammatory state of the injured tissues. Stiffness in the morning or after prolonged rest can be caused by fluid stasis.[16] Sleeping positions often result in decreased muscle contraction and diminished blood and lymph pressure. The metabolically active (injured) area gradually imbibes fluid, which increases osmotic pressure and decreases fluid drainage. This static state results in fluid congestion and causes regional hypoxia, decreased fluid drainage, and an accumulation of metabolites.[13, 14, 16, 34] These physiological changes create a chemical environment that results in peripheral and central axonal sensitization (i.e., chemical irritation; an increase in afferent neural activity because of the mechanical and chemical depolarization of the nervous terminals in the affected area).[3, 31] A sequelae of this increase in afferent input into the central nervous system is a concurrent increase in efferent output from the nervous system to the musculature, resulting in increased muscle guarding, palpable increased tissue tension, and the sensation of stiffness and soreness. Patients with injury or swelling caused by the degenerative process complain of the same sensations of stiffness and soreness after prolonged sitting or standing.

The patient who describes the morning as the best time of day, with no stiffness or soreness, only to find that the symptoms gradually increase as the day proceeds is probably mechanically, rather than chemically, stimulating nociceptors. Many of these patients do not possess the neuromuscular strength, coordination, and endurance to counterbalance the forces (compression, shear, tension, and torque) that are encountered as a result of gravity and movement during the activities of daily living. Consequently, prolonged or excessive stresses are placed on the passive support tissues of the musculoskeletal system, such as ligaments, articular cartilage, and bone, resulting in a decreased ability to transfer and attenuate forces. These patients mechanically stimulate the pain receptor system without detectable inflammation. This syndrome often is successfully managed with short-term physical therapy that emphasizes biomechanical counseling, postural awareness, and therapeutic exercise. In contrast, the patient who describes the morning as the worst time of day most often experiences pain as a result of a combination of chemical and mechanical stimulation of the nociceptive nervous system. This population of patients usually takes longer to respond to treatment because of the time constraints and limitations of tissue healing.[33]

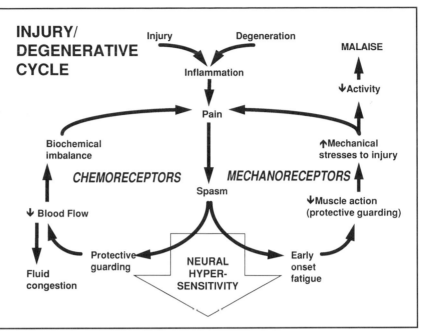

INJURY/ DEGENERATIVE CYCLE

Figure 5–1. Injury-degenerative cycle. This cycle represents the major components of the upper-quarter syndrome. The clinician should be cognizant of the interrelations of the mechanoreceptor and chemoreceptor afferent stimuli. The inability to attain painless activity often results in emotional disturbances broadly defined as malaise.

During the assessment, the clinician must be aware of the components of the injury-degeneration cycle (Fig. 5–1). This cycle depicts the relation between the mechanoreceptor and chemoreceptor afferent stimuli to the extent of the painful syndrome. After the assessment, the clinician must make a judgment as to the contribution of each portion of the cycle as it relates to the upper-quarter syndrome. This judgment represents the basis for developing the initial treatment goal. For example, if the findings suggest the existence of a significant inflammatory response and pain is experienced before or with the onset of resistance to passive or active movement, then the clinician visualizes the chemoceptor side of the cycle "spinning" faster than the mechanoreceptor side. The treatment is focused on activities that stimulate fluid dynamics and promote the healing potential.

Conversely, if prolonged antigravity postures and movements reproduce symptoms, the mechanoreceptor side is "spinning" faster than the chemoreceptor side. The therapeutic intervention includes such treatments as postural instruction, active exercise, and neuromuscular techniques to facilitate movement patterns that minimize nociceptive stresses.

In most cases, both sides of the cycle are spinning but at different rates. The importance of the cycle concept is the combined effect of each cycle on afferent input to the central nervous system. The ultimate effect is the influence on the sensitivity of the nervous system.[31] The primary goal of the treatment process is to reduce the sensitization of the afferent system by rapidly affecting the rate and extent of each side of the injury-degeneration cycle.

The assessment process explained in this chapter is based on a three-dimensional appreciation of the anatomy and the functional biomechanics. It recognizes the importance of involving the patient in the explanation of his or her painful syndrome and then emphasizing that he or she must assume responsibility in the management of the condition. The success of treatment depends on the quality of the communication between patient and clinician and the patient's willingness to assume as much responsibility as possible. The clinician's role is to guide the patient through a treatment process that consists of successfully identifying realistic short- and long-term goals. These goals are founded on the science of soft tissue healing. The clinician-patient relationship that totally relies on the clinician for management is destined for emotional, professional, and financial failure.

The assessment is best carried out in a properly lighted and comfortable environment. How the patient is greeted when entering the facility, the waiting time, and the temperature and lighting of the examination room are just a few factors that influence the clinician-patient interaction. Attention to such details sends an important message to the patient and can positively or negatively impact on the assessment and management process.

HISTORY

A complete, accurate history is essential to successful assessment and the development of a treatment plan. The history is designed to establish a clear understanding of the patient's pain pattern and perception of the problem, especially in regard to how the complaint is limiting function. The pain pattern consists of the intensity, frequency, and duration of the pain from the onset of the symptoms to the present. It is important that the patient recognize the parameters of the syndrome so that a pattern can be identified. Figure 5–2 shows an intake form used to record the information from the history.

The clinician should tailor the questions to elicit a description of the pain pattern without leading the patient. Most patients are unable to describe the subtle alterations of their painful syndrome and are not aware of the small changes as they occur. The realization that their syndrome has definition is important because the success of the treatment process depends on the patient's ability to recognize small changes in one or more of the pain pattern parameters.

The following information should be obtained from the history:

1. Longevity of symptoms
2. Position of initial pain or injury (if occurred)
3. Forces generated and positions of initial pain or injury (if occurred)
4. Graphical representations of the history from the onset to the present, daily behavior, and time and quality of sleep, which will determine the pain pattern

5. Description, site, and pattern of pain (pain drawing) since onset
6. List of the medications currently taken
7. Level of activity according to an activity scale
8. Level of stressors according to a stress scale
9. Patient's impression of problem

Once this information is obtained, the clinician must make a judgment as to the patient's level of comprehension so that the education process can effectively commence.

To develop an appreciation of the extent of the syndrome, the following questions need to be answered.

How Old Are You? What Is Your Occupation? Where Does It Hurt?

After a brief introduction, the first aspect of the history is the determination of the patient's age and occupation and the site of pain. The reason for determining the occupation is to recognize the forces and loads encountered during the workday. If the patient is working at home, the clinician should ask if the patient has children and the number and ages of the children. This provides information regarding the demands on the patient and the type of activities the patient is involved with at home.

This information and a determination of the site of pain are entered on the intake form (see Fig. 5–2). An accurate determination of the site of pain is important because it not only provides a point of discussion between clinician and patient, but also permits the clinician to begin to differentiate radicular from referred pain patterns.

Radicular pain occurs as a result of irritation to the nerve root complex and has a particular path and location (see Chapter 2). Radicular pain patterns become evident when the arm pain is worse or more distressing than the neck pain and can be felt in the absence of the neck pain. Referred pain often is the opposite; that is, the origin of the complaint is in the neck region, and as the pain intensifies, the pain migrates peripherally. Referred pain is pain that is felt away from the source. It is caused by an irritation of any of the innervated cervical spine tissues, is nondescript, and varies in location.[2] If radicular pain exists, the clinician should ask, "Is the arm pain worse than the neck pain? Or, does the pain pattern

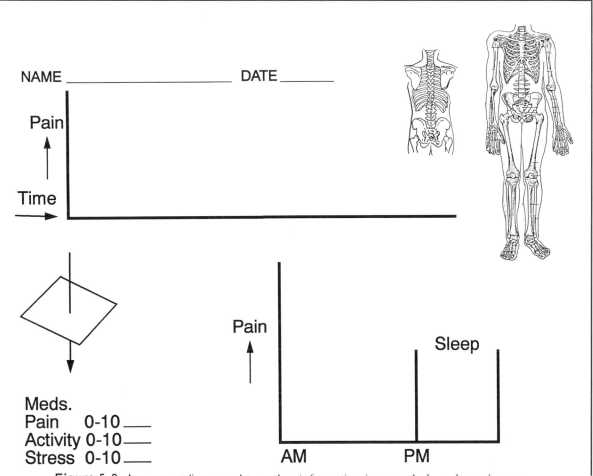

NAME _____ DATE _____

Pain

↑

Time

→

Meds.
Pain   0-10 ___
Activity 0-10 ___
Stress 0-10 ___

Pain

↑

Sleep

AM   PM

Figure 5–2. Assessment form used to gather information in an orderly and concise manner. Note the graphs (intensity of pain over time for the duration of the syndrome and for a 1-day period). Included on this form is a place to record a pain drawing, a square to record the range of motion that reproduces the familiar pain, and a place to record medication and to rank the activity scale (0–10) and stress scale (0–10).

begin in the neck and as the neck pain worsens, the pain into the arm and scapular region worsen?'' The answers to these questions often provide the clinician with information to help discern whether the pain is referred or radicular.

How Long Have You Had Neck Pain?

It is important to determine the time of the initial onset of the injury or whether the symptoms were insidious. This gives the clinician an idea of the time the body has had to adapt to the dysfunction. If the initial onset of the injury was 7 years ago and the patient has experienced five episodes of the similar pain, then the clinician can assume that adaptive changes have occurred and that these contribute to exacerbations of the syndrome. In contrast, if the onset of injury is recent without relief of pain, the clinician can make a judgment as to the current state of the healing process. The date of the initial onset is written in the bottom corner of the graph.

What Position Were You In Or What Were the Activities at the Time of Injury? Before the Initial Onset of Pain?

The clinician attempts to determine the positions and forces that were involved in the injury process or existed the day or hours before the initial experience of pain. This information permits the clinician to envision the position (mid or end range) of the tissues of the neck and the forces encountered (compression, torsion, shear, tension) during the painful syndrome. Were the tissues of the upper quarter at end range or mid range? Was the intensity of the forces generated during the initial episode enough to injure tissues? The answers to these questions provide the clinician with information regarding the extent of the injury and initial onset of pain.

How Many Episodes of Pain Have You Had Since the Onset, and How Long Has Each Lasted?

It often is useful to graph this information. The horizontal line of the graph represents time, and the vertical line represents the intensity of the pain. Once the initial onset has been defined and graphed, each subsequent episode should be similarly identified and graphed.

Graphing of the history should conclude by asking the patient about the current intensity of pain. This information can be gained by asking, ''If 0 is no pain and 10 is the worst pain you have experienced with this condition, what level of pain did you experience yesterday? What level of pain are you experiencing today?'' Graphically depicting the pain pattern provides information about the current pattern and whether the patient is in an exacerbation phase (enhanced pain) of the syndrome or the syndrome is improving.

Describe Your Pain

The next aspect of the history is to ask the patient to describe the pain. If the patient pauses, the clinician can assist by asking, ''Is the pain sharp, dull, aching, shooting, piercing, or . . .'' The patient usually picks up the conversation at this point. It may be difficult to describe the pain, but the patient should be encouraged to attempt to educate the clinician.

Once that information is recorded on the intake form (see Fig. 5–2), the characteristics of the pain can be discussed. If the clinician believes that the communication has been consistent and productive, then the pain pattern is graphed and approved by the patient. If the clinician thinks that there has been difficulty in communication or suspects malingering, symptom magnification, or illness behavior, the patient is asked to complete the pain drawing. Drawings that are excessive and nondescript may represent nonorganic signs of musculoskeletal disorders.[28] Nonorganic signs refer to pain behaviors and descriptions that do not follow normal anatomical and physiological guidelines. An abnormal pain drawing might be pain described in all aspects of the anatomy that does not follow expected dermatomes or myotomes. Using multiple symbols to illustrate pain on a body chart should also alert the clinician to the possibility of nonorganic signs.[6] These pain behaviors should be recognized by the clinician and placed in proper perspective as the assessment continues.

During the graphing of the history, the patient should be encouraged to modify or alter the graph to better define the syndrome. The clinician should encourage this assistance by the patient. Once the patient makes changes or attempts to clarify the graph to better depict the problem, the patient has begun to take an active role in improving his or her painful condition. Patients who refuse to communicate or are disinterested in the evaluation typically have poor treatment results.

One of the treatment goals is to maintain or increase the patient's activity level without increasing or exacerbating the painful syndrome. It is important that the patient confirm the accuracy of the graphic representation of the pain pattern because the graph represents a tool that can be revisited as the treatment process unfolds. It can be used effectively to set goals and depict patient progress.

Are You Stiffer and Sorer in the Morning or in the Evening?

Once the patient agrees that the drawing accurately depicts the pain pattern, the history can continue by graphing the daily pain behavior. As previously mentioned, the answer to this question is an important determinant of the existing inflammatory state of the tissue. This A.M./P.M./sleep graph (see Fig. 5–2) is used to document the status of the stiffness and soreness in the morning, track the intensity of the pain during the day, and determine the sleeping behavior at night. Figure 5–3 shows an example of this portion of the history.

Are You Sleeping Through the Night?

The last portion of the A.M./P.M. graph permits the clinician to document the patient's sleep pattern. It is common for a patient with neck and upper-quarter pain to have difficulty first getting comfortable at night and then, once asleep, completing the night without awakening. A common finding among patients with the diagnosis of fibromyalgia, a condition of nondescript spinal pain, is the inability to experience a deep, restful sleep.[9, 20, 27] Without restful sleep, a person, especially one who is experiencing pain, has diminished capability to cope with his or her painful syndrome.

It is important that the clinician associate the inability to gain control of a painful condition with the lack of quality sleep. The common medical treatment for a sleep deprivation condition is prescription medication. The logical next inquiry, however, is to ask the patient why he or she is not sleeping well. Such patients often have difficulty achieving the degree of relaxation required to gain restful sleep.

If the patient has not been sleeping well and has been unable to manage his or her neck problem, resolving this problem should be one of the first goals of the treatment process. Insomnia can be devastating and is not always tied to accumulated stressors. It is incorrect to associate all sleep disorders with the inability to manage stressors and to relax. The clinician needs to be aware of these circumstances and the role they play in the upper-quarter syndrome and in fibromyalgia. The diagnosis of fibromyalgia often presents as a syndrome accompanied by not only musculoskeletal tenderness, but biochemical changes and other manifestations as well.[4, 12, 15, 21, 25, 26, 32, 35]

Are You Taking Any Medications?

Most patients with musculoskeletal syndromes are prescribed medication either to decrease inflammation or to minimize pain. It is important that the clinician ascertain if the patient is taking medications, what medications are being taken, and if they are being taken as prescribed. Patients with neck pain commonly take nonsteroidal anti-inflammatory steroids. These medications inhibit prostaglandins, which are potent vasodilators. Other medications commonly used to treat neck pain are muscle relaxants and psychotherapeutic drugs for relaxation and sleep. The use of muscle relaxants for disorders that rely on protective guarding (spasm) appears to be counterproductive. Their use should be limited to the evening to improve the quality of sleep.

What Activities Make Your Pain Worse? What Activities Are Limited by This Problem?

These questions are directed toward understanding the limitations in activities of daily living and the occupational biomechanics that exacerbate the problem. It is important that the patient

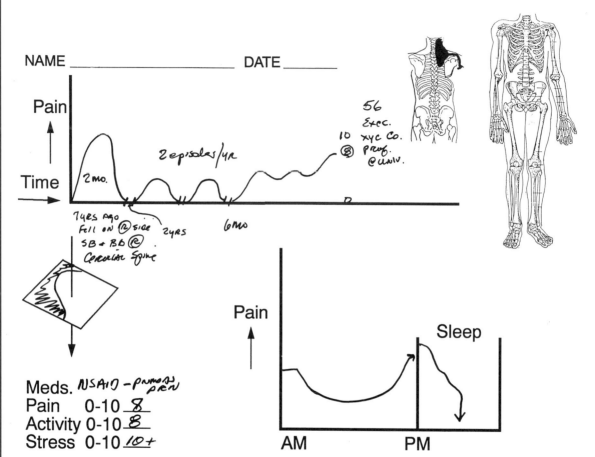

NAME _____ DATE _____

Pain

Time

2 mo.

2 episodes/yr

56
Exec.
10 xyc Co.
⑧ Prof.
@ Univ.

7yrs ago
Fell on ® side 2yrs
SB + BB ®
Cervical Spine

6mo

Meds. NSAID - pain med prn
Pain   0-10 _8_
Activity 0-10 _8_
Stress 0-10 _10+_

Pain

Sleep

AM   PM

Figure 5–3. The completed intake form seen in Figure 5–2. This patient, a 56-year-old executive, also is a college instructor. Seven years ago he fell on his right side, side bending and backward bending to the right on his cervical spine. He had right upper quadrant pain for a two-month period until the pain totally went away. For two years he had no problems whatsoever and then had two episodes of right neck and shoulder pain per year. Six months ago he was waxing his car and had gradual progressive increase in pain in the right side of the neck and shoulder and scapular region with occasional peripheralization to the mid arm. At no time in the last six months has he been pain free. He is at level 8 out of 10 on the pain scale. His pain is worse in the morning, decreases after movement, and progressively increases in proportion to activity. He has difficulty getting comfortable for sleep at night, but he sleeps until morning. He takes nonsteroidal anti-inflammatory medication and pain medication prn. He is at level 8 activity level (20 per cent of those things he wants to do he cannot do), and he is at 10 level stress. The patient notes a correlation between high stress levels and increased pain levels. This graph is one that can easily be read by other clinicians, is used at the end of the assessment to set goals, and is used at each visit to graphically monitor progress.

recognize the importance of analyzing each aspect of his or her life to assist the clinician in managing the syndrome. If the patient cannot explain or identify the activities (i.e., forces, positions, circumstances) that exacerbate the syndrome, then the clinician must help the patient to recognize a correlation between activity and pain.

How Active Are You?

The patient should be asked, "If 0 is bed rest and 10 is normal pre-pain activity, what is your activity level?" Another way to ask this question is, "What percentage of activities are you limited in doing because of this condition?" The answer to this question provides the clinician with two perspectives on the problem. The first is the patient's frustration level. The frustrated patient is angry that he or she has not been able to remain as active as he or she would like. The second perspective is related to the degree of disability perceived by the patient. For example, if the patient rates his or her activity level at 8, then the clinician should follow by asking, "Does this mean that this condition prevents you from doing 20 per cent of the activities you want to do?" If the response is yes, the question has probably been interpreted correctly. On the other hand, if the patient is confused, clarification is needed. The goal is to determine the extent to which the painful syndrome has affected physical activity by the answer and the manner in which the patient responds.

Have You Been Under a Great Deal of Stress?

The clinician can begin this discussion by saying, "Now that we have rated pain and activity, we would like to measure your level of stress. If 0 is no stress and 10 is major stress, what level of stress are you experiencing?"

As explained in Chapter 1, the accumulation of environmental and personal stressors can play a major role in the patient's ability to rest the tissues of the upper quarter and manage the problem. The patient may answer this question in one of two ways. The first is to state that he or she is not under an excessive amount of stress and then on reflection, offer "4 or 5." The other

general answer usually begins with a pause or frown. When this is the initial response, the clinician can respond by defining major stress. The purpose of this line of questioning is not to identify the stress or to invade a patient's personal life but to get the patient to recognize that there is a relation between stress and the perception of pain. Examples of significant stressors include recent illness or self or a family member, a death in the family, divorce, job loss, and job change. Once the patient begins to develop an appreciation of the relation between stress and the painful syndrome, he or she becomes more comfortable in describing the particular stressors. The question "Do you think that there is a direct relation between these high stress levels and your painful syndrome?" is an important one. The response usually is affirmative.

Special Questions

Certain questions should be asked of patients with cervicothoracic complaints.

Have you had dizzy spells? Patients who experience dizziness may have vestibular, circulatory, or sympathetic nervous system disturbance. If recognized by the patient as a concern, the clinician should consider diagnostic testing to rule out an underlying disorder.

Do you have tingling and numbness in both arms and hands or both legs? Do you have difficulty walking? Affirmative answers to these questions may signify spinal cord compression syndromes such as those caused by cervical spondylosis and would warrant further investigation.

If you experience headaches along with your neck pain, are they throbbing, irregular and unrelated to activity, or accompanied by blurred vision or nausea? If the patient can positively relate to this line of questioning, then migraine headaches must be ruled out.

Do you experience pain or numbness in or about your face? Patients who can relate to this type of referral pattern into the face and temporomandibular joint may have neuralgia or neuritis associated with distributions of the peripheral or cranial nerves. This condition should be specifically assessed to rule out other disorders.[4]

What do you think is the basis of your problem? It is important that the patient be given an opportunity to express his or her viewpoint. This type of question indicates that the clinician is going to rely on the patient's attention and assistance and that the patient's perception of the problem is crucial. Instead of a come-to-my-office-and-let-me-take-care-of-your-problem approach, the successful clinician projects the philosophy of "come to my office and allow me to assist you in taking care of your problem." The patient must take responsibility for the condition and for his or her overall health.

STANDING EXAMINATION

Inspection

The frontal and sagittal planes are inspected to observe the postural relations between the head,

Table 5–1. Standing Examination
Inspection
Structure (sagittal/frontal plane) cervical
Structure frontal (lumbopelvic)
Gross movement testing of upper extremities
Active humeral flexion
Active humeral abduction—scapulohumeral rhythm

neck, shoulder complex, and abdominal wall mechanism (Table 5–1). The relations between these regions in the static posture provide information regarding the compression, tension, and shear stresses encountered by the specialized connective tissues of the upper quarter (see Chapter 1).

Frontal plane inspection also provides information regarding the lumbopelvic base, which

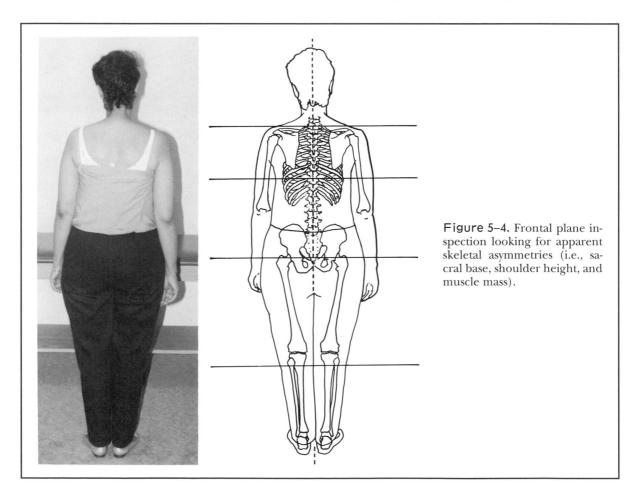

Figure 5–4. Frontal plane inspection looking for apparent skeletal asymmetries (i.e., sacral base, shoulder height, and muscle mass).

can be a factor in force attenuation of the upper quarter (Fig. 5–4). The lumbopelvic base can be quickly assessed by comparing the levels of the iliac crests, posterior superior iliac spines, anterior superior iliac spines, and greater trochanters (Fig. 5–5).[22] Frontal plane asymmetry can influence the mechanics of the upper quarter in certain body types, especially the nonadapting musculoskeletal system that poorly attenuates the shock and forces of weight bearing and movement. If the patient's musculoskeletal system ineffectively attenuates forces, the effects of an asymmetrical frontal plane probably will be detected lower in the spine and may not play a significant role in an upper-quarter problem. Up-per-quarter assessments, however, should begin with a frontal plane structural screen.[10] Continued frontal plane observations include the positions of the scapulae, height of the shoulders, carrying angle of the elbows, and presence of a list in the cervical spine. Atrophy or hypertrophy of the musculature related to the cervical spine or shoulder girdle should also be noted at this time.

The inspection continues by observing overall postural alignment. The patient's assumed posture often is established by the central nervous system as a means to minimize nociceptive input. The clinician must recognize this neurophysiological influence and then decide which aspect

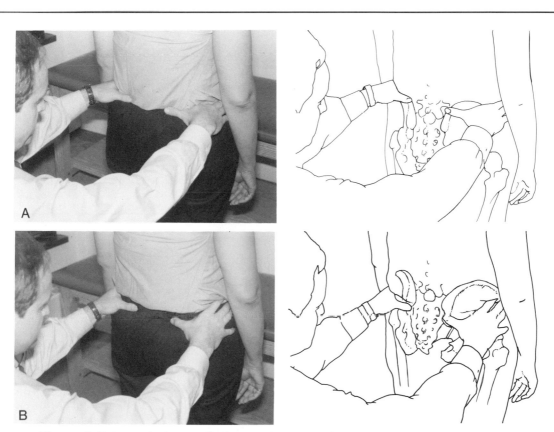

Figure 5–5. Frontal plane palpation to determine the status of the sacral base. Four anatomical landmarks are palpated to establish this relationship. *A,* Palpation of iliac crest. *B,* Palpation of posterior superior iliac crest (PSIS).

Illustration continued on following page

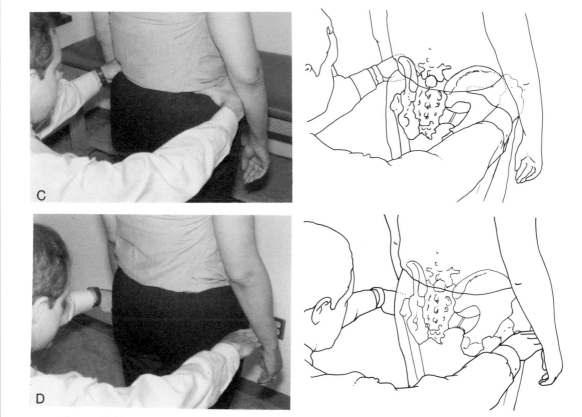

Figure 5–5 *Continued C,* Palpation of anterior superior iliac crest (ASIS). *D,* Palpation of greater trochanters.

of the postural change must be addressed in the treatment process. The decision is made by relating the assessment findings to the postural changes noted.

Postural inspection in the sagittal plane follows (Fig. 5–6). This observation is important because it also informs the clinician as to how the upper quarter is attenuating forces and how the sagittal plane posture might be affecting movement.

The sagittal plane of our antigravity posture is controlled in part by the abdominal wall musculature, and the influence of the abdominal wall on the upper quarter should be understood. If the abdominal wall is weak and lengthens, the chest descends, resulting in a forward-bending moment at the thoracic spine (Fig. 5–7). This moves the weight line of the upper trunk anteriorly.

As a result of abdominal wall and thorax changes, the chest descends and the scapula migrates forward around the rib cage, approximating the clavicle to the first rib. The humerus assumes a more internally rotated position. The head and neck are brought forward, and to keep the eyes horizontal, the patient must extend the occiput. This not only alters the cervical lordosis and the weight-bearing pattern of the apophyseal joints, but also increases the activity of the extensor muscles, especially the suboccipital muscles. The abdominal wall thus plays a significant role in the mechanics of upper-quarter posture.

The weakness and increased length of the abdominal wall also negate the effect of the hydraulic cylinder created by the diaphragm and pelvic floor muscles.[11] This loss of abdominal muscle function changes the way in which the forces of gravity and movement attenuate throughout the spine.

Restoring the strength and endurance of the abdominal muscles and balancing the anterior and posterior scapular muscles help to secure a more efficient carrying position for the head, neck, and shoulders and commonly are used as the basis of treatment for many cervical conditions. Strengthening of the abdominal wall should be performed without compromising the neck. After inspection, the clinician proceeds with gross movement testing.

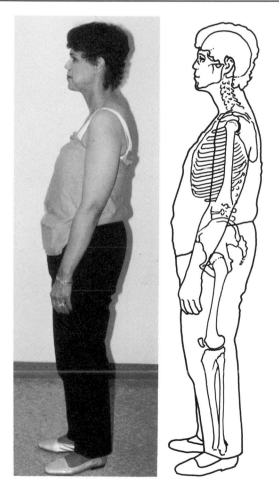

Figure 5–6. Inspection is also done in the sagittal plane. One should recognize the forward-head, rounded-shoulder posture, which is mainly a result of the integrity of the abdominal wall and hip joints.

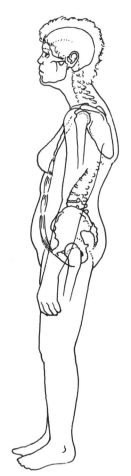

Figure 5–7. Forward-head, rounded-shouldered posture from a sagittal view showing the result of a lengthened abdominal wall and alterations of the posture, causing the chest wall to migrate downward. Note the forward head, increased cervical lordosis, round shoulders, internally rotated humerus, and kyphotic posture.

Gross Movement Testing

While the clinician stands behind the patient, the patient is asked to raise the arms in front of the body and over the head (Fig. 5–8*A*) and then out and away from the body as far as possible (Fig. 5–8*B*). These motions are repeated so that

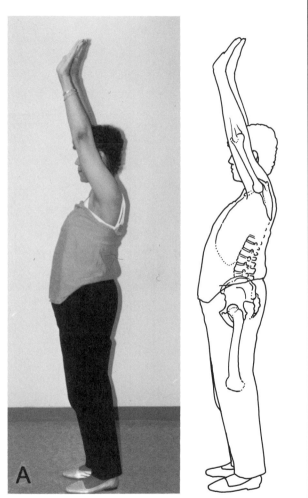

Figure 5–8. *A,* The patient is asked to actively forward elevate. Here the evaluator is looking for glenohumeral rhythm and symmetrical motion.

Illustration continued on following page

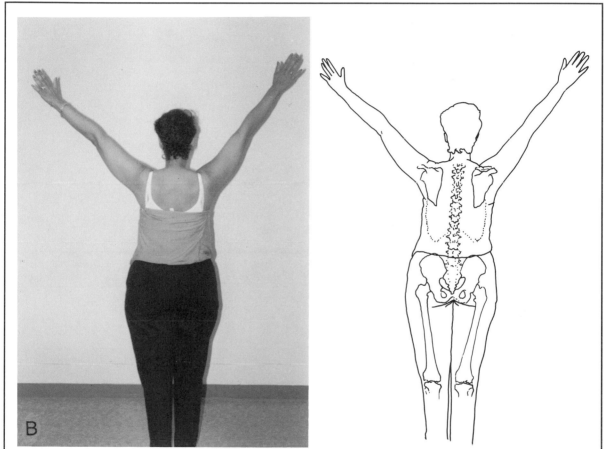

Figure 5-8. *Continued B,* The patient is asked to actively abduct. Here the evaluator is looking for glenohumeral rhythm and symmetrical motion.

the clinician can ascertain the movement patterns of the glenohumeral, scapulothoracic, and cervicothoracic regions. Full active shoulder flexion requires lower cervical and thoracic spinal extension; a limitation in the end ranges of shoulder movement may be caused by pain from the extension and compression forces in the cervicothoracic spine.

If there is asymmetry in movement, especially in movement of the scapulae, the serratus anterior and other scapular muscles should be tested. Manual muscle testing or a wall push-up maneuver in the standing position can be done to assess serratus anterior muscle strength.[17] The patient is asked to stand about 16 inches from a wall and then lean into it. The clinician closely observes the scapulae as the patient pushes against the wall. Weakness is represented by "winging" of the scapula or failure to maintain the position of the scapula against the rib cage.

SITTING EXAMINATION

The patient is then asked to sit on the edge of the treatment table. This position permits the clinician to observe the quality and range of active cervical motion, perform overpressure testing to the tissues of the neck, conduct a strength screen by means of manual muscle testing (Table 5–2), and complete the neurological screen (Table 5–3). The sitting position allows the information to be gained with the head and neck in the upright antigravity position.

Active Range of Motion—Rotation

The patient is asked to actively rotate the cervical spine first to the right (Fig. 5–9A) and then to the left (Fig. 5–9B) while the clinician observes the total range to each side, fluidity of motion, and whether pain is reproduced. The quality of movement is determined in part by how smooth the motion is, catches during the motion, and the degree of substitution or muscle guarding that occurs.

Table 5–2. Sitting Examination

Active range of motion
Rotation: End-range testing
  Active cervical rotation to the right
  Active cervical rotation to the left
  Active cervical rotation to the right
  Overpressure (rotation and rotation and backward bending)
  Active cervical rotation to the left
  Overpressure (rotation and rotation and backward bending)
Forward bending: End-range testing
  Active cervical forward bending
  Active cervical forward bending
    Overpressure toward side bending to the right
    Overpressure toward side bending to the left
Backward bending: End-range testing
  Active cervical backward bending
  Active cervical backward bending
    Overpressure in backward bending
    Overpressure in backward bending and side bending to the right
    Overpressure in backward bending and side bending to the left
Combination backward bending-side bending: End-range testing
Passive humeral motion: (flexion, abduction, rotation)
Manual strength screening
  Bilateral humeral flexion at 90 degrees of flexion
  Bilateral humeral abduction at 90 degrees of abduction
  Arms at side, elbows flexed, to test bilateral external rotators

Table 5–3. Neurological Screen

Neurological Screening: Reflexes
  C5 Biceps brachii
  C6 Brachioradialis
  C7 Triceps
Neurological Screening: Myotomes
  C5 Deltoid, biceps
  C6 Biceps, wrist extensors
  C7 Triceps, wrist flexors
  C8 Extensor pollicus longus, finger flexors
  T1 Interossei, abductor digiti minimi
Neurological Screening: Dermatomes
  C5 Lateral brachium
  C6 Lateral antibrachium, thumb, first finger
  C7 Middle finger ½ ring finger, mid palm
  C8 ½ ring finger, little finger, medial antibrachium
  T1 Medial elbow region
Neural Tension Tests
  Thoracic outlet
  Median nerve tension
  Ulnar nerve tension

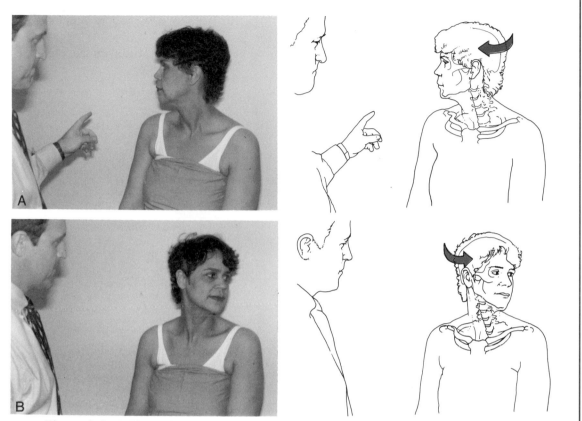

Figure 5–9. *A*, The patient is asked to actively rotate the head to the right. *B*, The patient is asked to actively rotate the head and neck to the left.

End-Range Testing: Rotation and Combined Movements

After active rotation has been observed, the patient is asked to repeat the motions. Overpressure in rotation is imparted by way of the occiput, using the occiput and temporal region of the skull as hand placements and pressure points (Fig. 5–10*A*).

The clinician's right elbow is placed just anterior to the left shoulder to block rotation of the thoracic spine during the overpressure test to the cervical spine. If this stabilization does not occur, a false interpretation of cervical spine rotation results because of rotation of the trunk. From this overpressure position, the clinician can drop his or her right hand down to the mid cervical spine.

This area is used as a fulcrum over which forces of backward bending and backward bending with side bending is performed.

Using the left hand, a backward bending force of the cervical spine over the clinician's fixed right hand can be carried out. This position permits the clinician to focus the forces of backward bending and backward bending with right side bending toward the clinician's right (fixated) hand. The force applied by the fixating hand is in a superior and anterior direction, which parallels the plane of the articular surfaces of the apophyseal joint of the midcervical vertebrae (Fig. 5–11).

The clinician should visualize creating a fixating force to the inferior vertebrae of the functional unit while the left hand simultaneously imparts a force resulting in backward bending and then backward bending with right side bending. This convergence of forces creates a localized compression force to the apophyseal joint surfaces and a tensile force to the joint capsule and support tissues on both sides of the vertebrae.

The clinician should assess whether pain is elicited before, simultaneously with, or after the resistance of overpressure is encountered.[7] If the pain is provoked before resistance, then the state of the tissue is acute and easily irritated. If pain is provoked at the point at which resistance or tightness is perceived, the clinician can conclude that the tissue can withstand more forces of activity and weight bearing without exacerbation. If pain is perceived after resistance is encountered, the patient is a candidate for a more active rehabilitation program without the chance for reinjury.

Information provided by end-range testing with overpressure can help the clinician determine the state of irritation of the tissues and whether the injury or lesion is at or above the

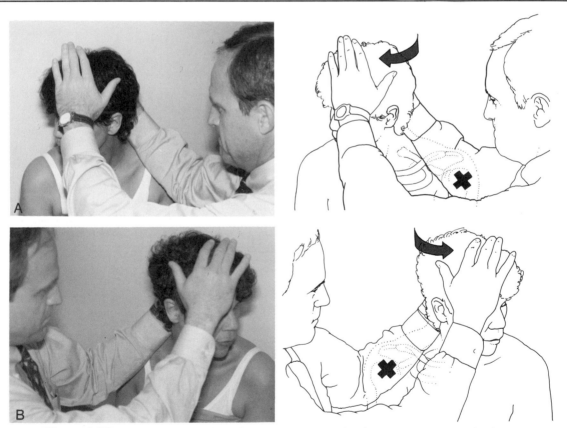

Figure 5–10. *A,* Overpressure in right rotation is done by the examiner. Note the forces imparted to the cranium at the forehead and lateral occipital regions. The examiner's right elbow is anterior to the patient's left shoulder to assure that the motion is centered or focused at the cervical spine. *B,* Overpressure in left rotation is done by the examiner. Note the forces imparted to the cranium at the forehead and lateral occipital regions. The examiner's left elbow is anterior to the patient's right shoulder to ensure that the motion is centered or focused at the cervical spine.

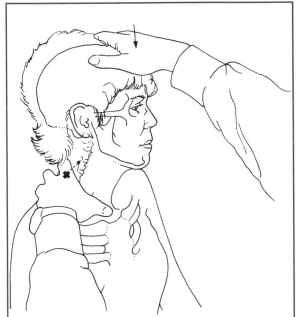

Figure 5–11. Forces imparted to the neck in the sitting examination using a fixated hand as a force from below upward and the hand on the occiput as the force from above downward.

nician to examine all the tissues at and above the fixation point, thus allowing for specific regions of the cervical spine to be evaluated.

The patient is then asked to rotate to the left, and the opposite hand position is used on the occiput with fixation of the right shoulder so that overpressure in left cervical rotation can be evaluated (Fig. 5–10*B*). The clinician then moves the left hand inferiorly to the midcervical spine, and rotation and backward bending with overpressure follow.

The clinician imparts forces to the cervical spine in an attempt to exacerbate the familiar symptom. Once the symptoms are reproduced, the clinician analyzes the forces as they traverse the spine. It is important to reproduce the patient's familiar symptom in an antigravity position not only so the clinician can use this information as a guide for treatment, but also as a means to analyze whether the response to these same forces and positions can be substantiated in the supine and prone positions.

Active Range-of-Motion and End-Range Testing: Forward Bending and Combined Movements

The sitting examination continues by asking the patient to forward bend the head and neck as far as possible (Fig. 5–12). This motion should be noted carefully to be sure that the motion is occurring in the cervical spine and is not simply a gross movement of the thoracic spine. Likewise,

level of the fixated hand. The clinician's right hand can then be moved to a lower region of the cervical spine, and a backward-bending overpressure again takes place at the fixated hand. This merely changes the fulcrum and permits the cli-

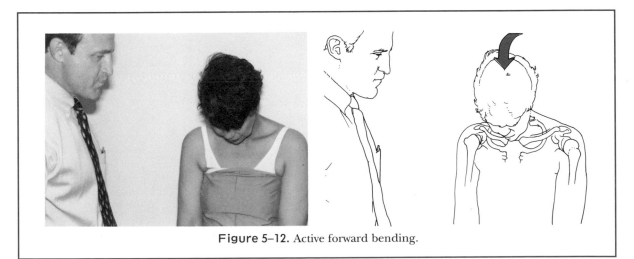

Figure 5–12. Active forward bending.

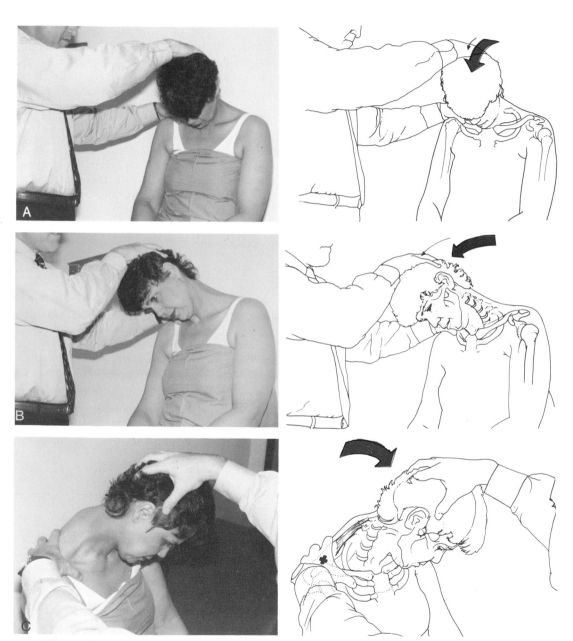

Figure 5–13. *A*, Active forward bending with overpressure. *B*, Active forward bending and side bending to the right with overpressure. The examiner causes a contract-relax and stretch to the left posterior musculature, mainly that of the posterior scalene, semispinalis surfaces, and levator scapulae. *C*, Active forward bending and side bending to the left with overpressure imparting a tensile force to these tissues.

the clinician should be cognizant of the difference between anterior sagittal rotation of the cervical vertebrae (true cervical flexion) and simply bringing the neck in a forward direction.

The clinician creates overpressure in forward bending by placing the left hand on the patient's right shoulder to allow for stabilization of the trunk and uses the right hand to direct tensile forces to the tissues on the posterior aspect of the cervical spine (Fig. 5–13A). The overpressure is carried out in a manner that attempts to increase the anterior sagittal rotation of the cervical spine.

The patient is then asked to forward bend and right-side bend the head and neck (Fig. 5–13B). The response to overpressure from this position is assessed. The examination continues with the patient combining the movements of forward bending and side bending to the left. The clinician again places a tensile force on the posterolateral tissues and attempts to reproduce the familiar symptom (Fig. 5–13C).

While performing these tests in the forward-bending quadrants, it is important that the clinician be able to visualize the forces imparted into and through the tissues of the upper quarter as the movement takes place. For example, forward bending with side bending to the right with overpressure creates compression at the right anterior corner of the intervertebral disc and the right apophyseal joint. From those two points, tissues located posteriorly and on the left side of the cervical spine are placed in varying degrees of tension. A three-dimensional appreciation of functional anatomy is critical to determining the forces and positions that exacerbate the familiar symptoms.

Active Range-of-Motion and End-Range Testing: Backward Bending and Combined Movements

The patient is asked to look upward to actively backward bend the cervical spine and then to repeat this motion using combined movements of extension and side bending (Fig. 5–14). If the patient complains of dizziness, light-headedness, or nausea or the clinician observes nystagmus during these motions, further evaluation is required. The clinician should screen for a possible compromise of the vertebral artery. Vertebral artery assessment is carried out from the supine position with the head and neck extended, rotated, and placed in full side bending. This combined position assesses vertebral artery patency. If similar findings of nystagmus and lapse of consciousness are observed, the clinician should seek further diagnostic evaluation to rule out potentially dangerous conditions that involve the vertebral arteries.[19]

After the patient performs sagittal plane extension and then the extension quadrant ranges of motion, the clinician places the right palm on

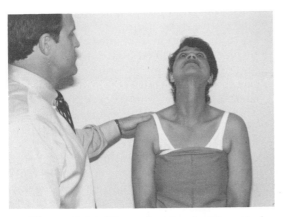
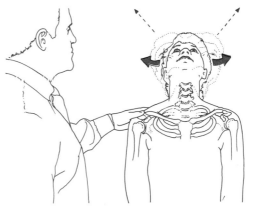

Figure 5–14. The patient is asked to actively extend and then to look up into each of the corners, first to the right and then to the left.

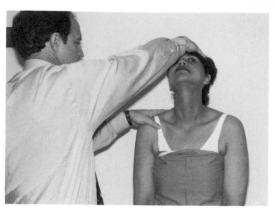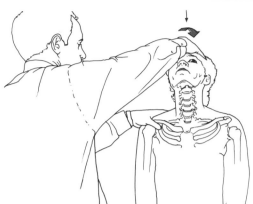

Figure 5–15. Overpressure and backward bending. Forces are imparted to the frontal aspect of the cranium, and one can visualize a 50/50 weight-bearing relation of the apophyseal joints, especially at the transition of the cervical and thoracic regions.

the patient's forehead and gently directs a superior-to-inferior force through the cervical spine (Fig. 5–15). Depending on how the overpressure is applied, the forces can be varied to load the cervical spine tissues in varying amounts of compression or tension.

One can visualize the forces that are generated to both apophyseal joints symmetrically during backward bending with overpressure. The force is generated through the occiput continuing down into and through the cervical spine. The position and forces cause the inferior articulating process to compress the joint surfaces, placing a tensile force on the apophyseal joint capsules as the inferior articulating process moves inferiorly and posteriorly on the superior articulating process. The force also compresses the posterior aspect of the intervertebral disc and places a tensile stress on the anterior longitudinal ligament and soft tissues anterior to the cervical vertebrae.

The overpressure force initially results in a posterior shear at the vertebral body–intervertebral disc as the compressive force between the articular surfaces is increased. Continued overpressure can also accentuate the cervical lordosis, in which case an anterior shear force results at the apex of

the convexity. If tissues designed to counter these forces are injured and unable to tolerate these stresses, pain is provoked.

The patient is then asked to backward bend and side bend to the right as the clinician generates gentle overpressure (Fig. 5–16A). This position results in moving the weight line or center of pressure from a posterior central position to a more posterior lateral position. The forces converge into the right posterior lateral articular surface of the right apophyseal joint. Although similar to the rotation and side-bending examination technique described above, the difference is the end-range position in which overpressure is applied. The forces are directed to the spine in a similar position but from different directions. The clinician should recognize at which point the pain is elicited—before, with, or after the resistance sensed with overpressure.

The examination continues by backward bending and side bending to the left in a similar manner and with the application of overpressure. This position assesses the weight-bearing function of the left side of the cervical spine (Fig. 5–16B).

Both the upper and the lower cervical spine are examined with these tests. However, the up-
Text continued on page 144

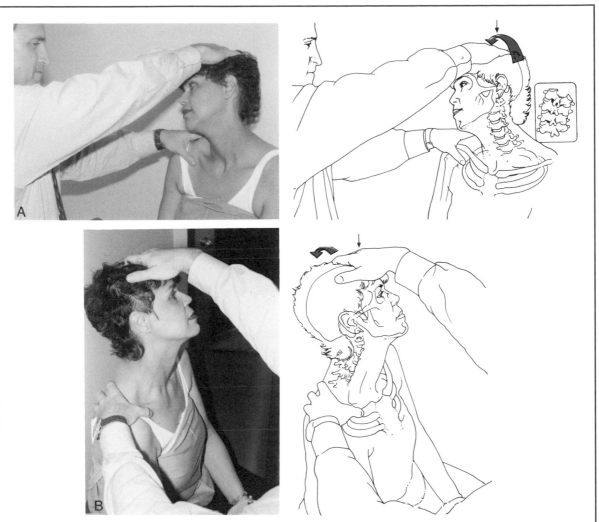

Figure 5–16. *A*, The patient's head is backward bent and side bent to the right with a direct vertical pressure imparted to the anterior left aspect of the patient's cranium. The clinician should be able to visualize a closed pack position or the right posterior aspect of the cervical spine, creating compression and shear. *B*, The patient's head is backward bent and side bent to the left with a direct vertical pressure imparted to the anterior right aspect of the patient's cranium. Note the examiner's left hand placement on the patient's right shoulder.

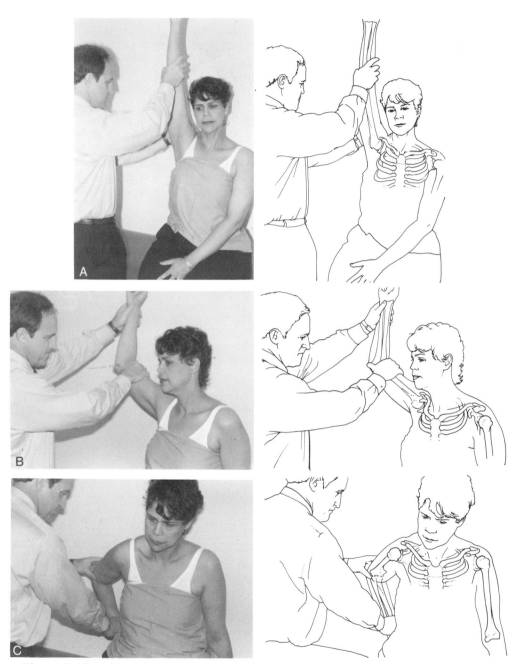

Figure 5–17. *A,* Passive right humeral flexion. *B,* Passive right humeral flexion, abduction, external rotation. *C,* Passive right humeral extension, internal rotation.

Illustration continued on following page

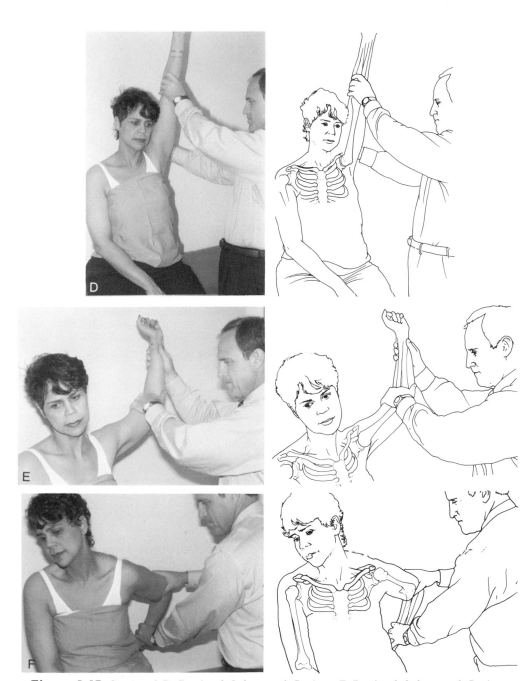

Figure 5–17 *Continued D,* Passive left humeral flexion. *E,* Passive left humeral flexion, abduction, external rotation. *F,* Passive left humeral extension, internal rotation.

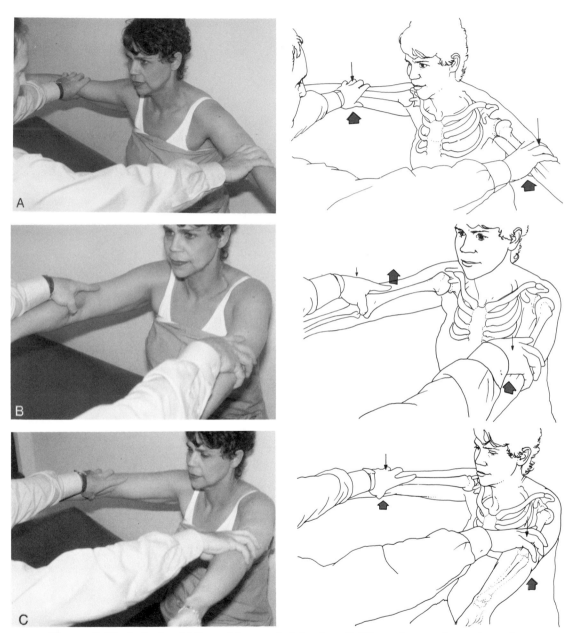

Figure 5–18. *A,* Resisted bilateral humeral abduction. *B,* Bilateral manual muscle testing of humeral flexion. *C,* Manual resistance testing with both humerus flexed, slightly adducted and internally rotated (supraspinatus test).

Illustration continued on following page

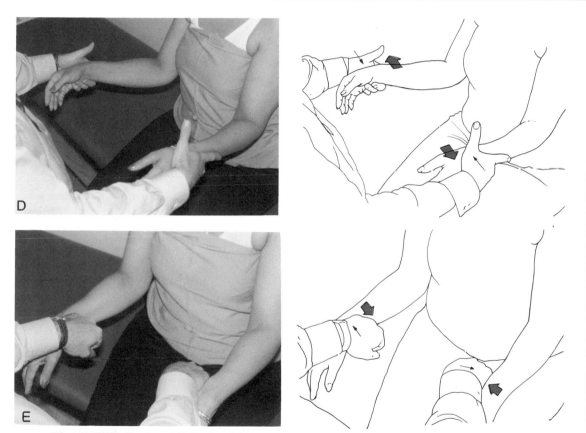

Figure 5-18 *Continued D*, Resisted humeral external rotation with humerus adducted and elbows at 90-degree flexion test. *E*, Resisted internal rotation with humerus adducted and elbows at 90-degree flexion test.

per cervical and lower cervical spine carry out different functions because of their specialized anatomy (see Chapter 4). Each area has different movement patterns, but both regions are composed of tissues that must possess load-bearing and transferring capabilities. A judgment as to the involvement of the upper cervical spine can be made, depending on the location and quickness of onset of pain (i.e., the forces of the assessment pass through the upper cervical spine first). A patient with injury to the upper cervical tissues experiences familiar pain early in the introduction of the evaluation forces.

In addition, movements isolated to the upper cervical spine can be assessed by positioning the lower cervical spine in end range of side bending. This position maintains the position of the lower cervical spine in side bending and rotation to the same side. By maintaining this position of the lower cervical spine and then turning the head in the opposite direction, motion between the atlas and axis is assessed. Again, the clinician is looking for the total range of movement to the right and left, the ease with which the motion occurs, and whether pain is reproduced. This region is further evaluated in the supine lying portion of the evaluation.

At this point in the assessment process, the clinician should have reproduced the familiar complaint (symptom) if the injury or lesion is in the cervical spine. This examination scheme permits the clinician to then seek assessment matches. Matches refer to the similarities of forces and positions that provoke symptoms in both a weight-bearing and a non–weight-bearing position. It is important to develop these matches to determine the consistency of patient information and ascertain the ease with which the pain is provoked. This information directs the treatment process. If a match is developed, the patient probably has an activity-related spinal disorder. If a match cannot be determined, then a more complex problem can be suspected, including referred pain from other musculoskeletal regions or visceral structures.

During the assessment, the clinician must be able to envision the anatomy moving in three dimensions to assess those forces and positions that reproduce the familiar symptoms (nociceptive biomechanics). This information represents the basis of the treatment process. The goal of

treatment is to assist the patient in minimizing the noxious stimuli so that prompt and complete healing can take place.

The examination continues by assessing the peripheral tissues of the upper quarter to determine the extent of their involvement and to establish the manner in which the forces are generated into and through the cervical spine from the periphery.

Screening the Shoulder Girdle

With the patient seated, the clinician can screen the shoulder complex by performing passive humeral flexion, abduction, external rotation, extension, internal rotation, and the combined movement of flexion to 90 degrees with horizontal adduction (impingement position; Fig. 5–17). It is quite common to find a relation between dysfunction of the scapulohumeral region and cervical pain, especially with the shoulder impingement syndrome associated with the forward-head posture.

If pain is reproduced in the neck when testing the shoulder, further assessment of the shoulder girdle is indicated. If pain is reproduced in the shoulder with these tests, then treatment designed to minimize the inflammatory process of these tissues is indicated. If one has a shoulder problem that results in substitution of muscle function, the cervical spine tissue can be compromised. Manual muscle testing of the shoulder complex can then be performed. Figure 5–18 shows a manual muscle test of the upper quarter.

Neurological Screening

The sitting examination continues by assessing nervous system function by means of reflex testing, myotome testing, sensory testing, and neural complex tension testing. The neurological screen is detailed in Table 5–3. This screen is used to determine the conduction (reflexes, myotomes, dermatomes) and inflammation (neural tension) of the neural tissues of the upper quarter.

Figure 5–19 shows the techniques for reflex testing of the upper quarter. The reflexes are reviewed in Chapter 2. If asymmetry (hyperreflexia or hyporeflexia) is observed, then the finding on the side of the neck complaint should be correlated to disturbed neural conduction, if pos-

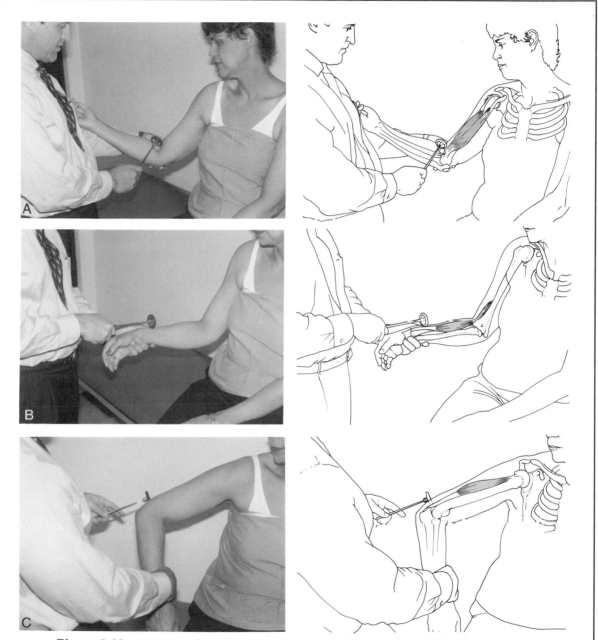

Figure 5–19. *A*, Testing of the C5 reflex (bicep brachii). *B*, Testing of C6 reflex (brachioradialis). *C*, Testing of the C7 reflex (triceps).

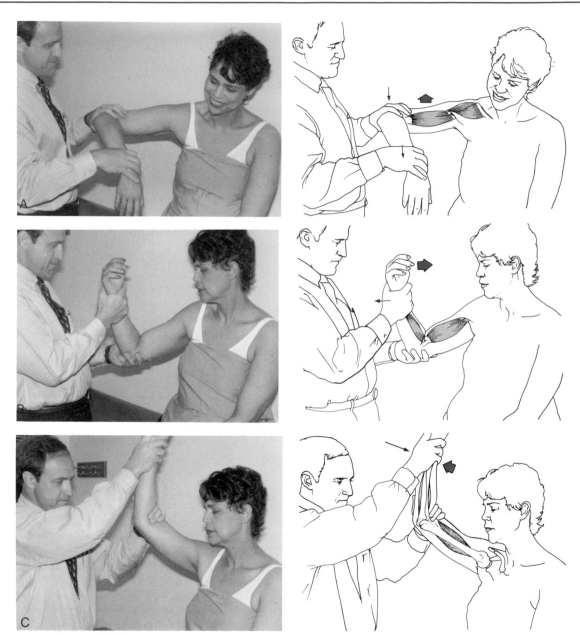

Figure 5–20. *A,* Manual muscle testing C5-6 deltoid and biceps. *B,* Manual muscle testing of C6 biceps and wrist extensors. *C,* Manual muscle testing of C7 triceps and wrist flexors.

Illustration continued on following page

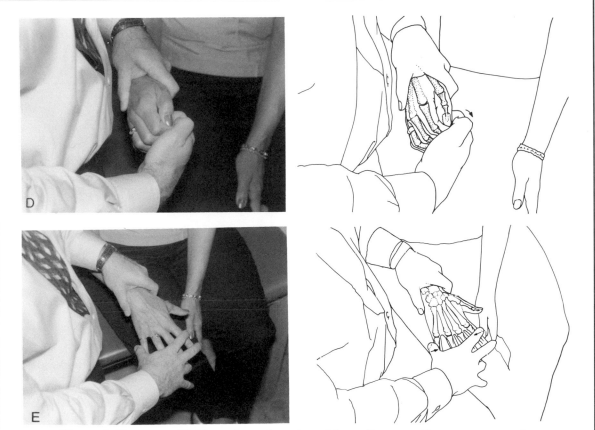

Figure 5–20 *Continued D*, Manual muscle testing of finger flexors and interosseous muscles (C8). *E*, Manual muscle testing of the digiti minimi T1.

sible. For example, if a patient has right-sided neck pain, increased pain or peripheralization of pain with extension and side bending to the right, and hyporeflexia of the right upper extremity, an axonal conduction disturbance can be suspected.

Figure 5–20 shows the techniques for evaluating myotomes of the upper quarter.[18] Normal findings would be an absence of pain and normal muscle strength with resisted testing. An abnormal neural screen would be muscle weakness but no reproduction of familiar pain. The provocation of pain with resisted tests suggests that contractile tissues and/or those tissues with which the contractile elements are related are injured.

The next aspect of the neurological screen is to assess cutaneous sensation. Figure 5–21 shows the dermatomal arrangement of the upper quarter. During the neurological assessment, the sensory innervation needs to be carefully screened to determine normal afferent axonal conduction. Circumferentially assessing cutaneous sensation is advocated to optimally compare upper-extremity dermatomes. This is shown in Figure 5–22.

The last aspect of the neurological screen is to assess the tensile capacity of the brachial plexus, using selected peripheral nerves, such as the median (Fig. 5–23) and the ulnar (Fig. 5–24).[5] These neural tension tests are described in Chapter 2.

Neurovascular compression of the brachial plexus and subclavian vessels can also be assessed

Text continued on page 152

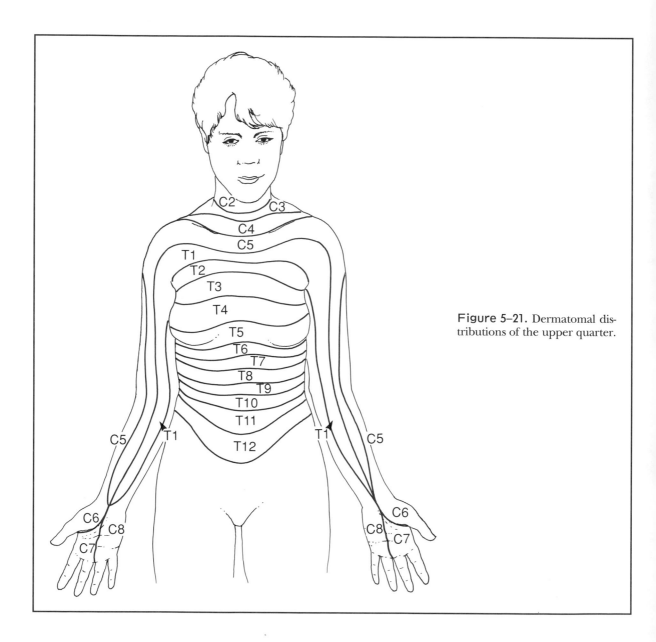

Figure 5–21. Dermatomal distributions of the upper quarter.

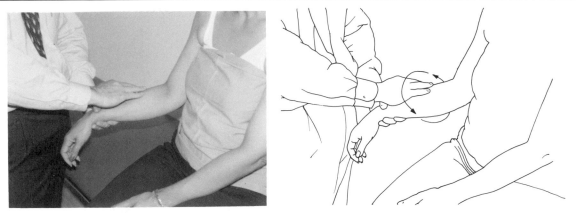

Figure 5–22. Sensory testing in a circular manner of the forearm, which is a sensory screen for the cervical nerve roots.

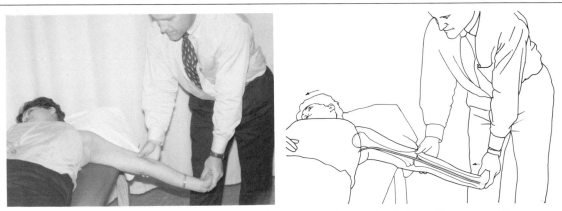

Figure 5–23. Positioning the patient to increase tension to the left median nerve. The head and neck are side bent to the right and the right humerus is abducted and externally rotated. The left elbow is fully extended. The left wrist and fingers are fully extended.

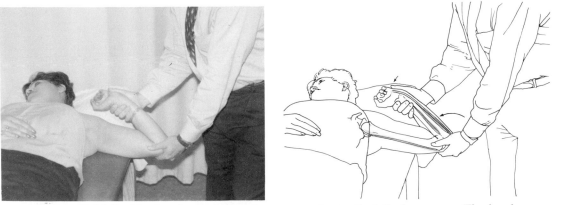

Figure 5–24. Positioning the patient to increase tension to the left ulnar nerve. The head and neck are side bent to the right and the left humerus is abducted. The left elbow is fully flexed, and the left wrist is radially deviated.

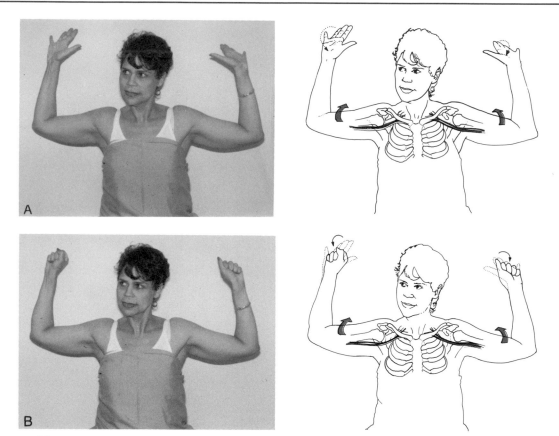

Figure 5–25. Thoracic outlet test. The patient is asked to flex, abduct, and externally rotate both arms. The clinician can visualize the forces imparted to the neurovascular bundle within the thoracic outlet in this position. The instruction to the patient is to open and close the hands as fast as possible. A positive finding is a change in the coordination of the movement or a decrease in the smoothness of function. This represents a tension and a compromise in blood flow, causing disturbance in neural conduction.

Figure 5–26. Adson test. This test is designed to direct tension and compression to the neurovascular bundle of the brachial plexus. These forces assimilate those of thoracic outlet syndrome (neurovascular compression syndrome). The example is performed on the right side. The examiner first palpates the radial pulse on the patient's right arm. The goal of the test is to obliterate the radial pulse by positioning the arm and chest to maximally assimilate those forces of a narrowed thoracic outlet. As the clinician continues to palpate the right radial pulse, the patient's right arm is extended and externally rotated. The patient is asked to rotate the head to the right and take a deep breath. Humeral extension and external rotation place a tensile force to the brachial plexus and related blood vessels. Cervical rotation to the right draws the anterior scalene back into the neurovascular bundle, creating a compression and tensile force to the tissues, and then inspiration raises the first rib up into the bundle, theoretically maximizing the compression force. A positive finding is the obliteration of the radial pulse, raising the suspicion of thoracic outlet syndrome.

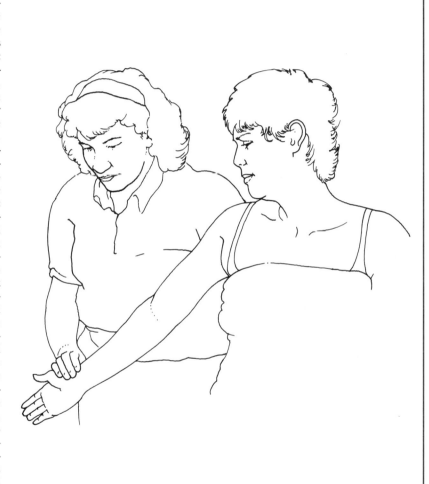

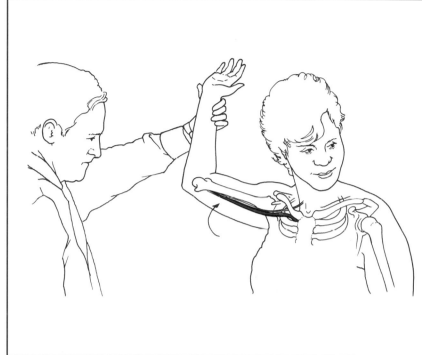

Figure 5–27. Allen test. This test is another designed to assess the tensile capability of the brachial plexus. If the examiner is to test the right plexus, the radial pulse is first assessed at the right wrist. The patient is asked to side bend to the left and rotate to the left. This position places a tensile force to the plexus. The examiner, while maintaining a read on the radial pulse, passively flexes, abducts, and externally rotates the right arm. The right elbow is extended, and the entire right upper extremity is extended. This position places the maximum stretch on the tissues of the brachial plexus. A positive finding is an obliteration of the radial pulse, indicating a compromise to the neurovascular bundle.

at this point in the examination (Fig. 5–25). Two of the more common tests that assess the presence of neurovascular compression syndrome (thoracic outlet) are the Adson test (Fig. 5–26) and the Allen test (Fig. 5–27). Although these tests are based on sound anatomical and biomechanical principles, the findings are difficult to reproduce and often yield false-positive results.

SUPINE LYING EXAMINATION

Palpation

The patient is asked to lie supine so that further examination of the upper quarter and the development of matches can take place (Table 5–4). This part of the examination begins with palpation. Palpation is used to assess the tissue tension sense or resting state of the muscle tissues, swelling, and the ease in reproducing pain with pressure. Any of these findings suggests tissue pathology or abnormality.

Table 5–4. Supine Lying Examination

Palpation
  Occiput and suboccipital region
  Identify C2 spinous process
  One fingerbreadth lateral—articular pillars
  Lateral cervical muscular
Active cervical extension and flexion
Passive rotation/side bending: End-range testing
  Passive rotation to the right—overpressure
  Passive rotation to the left—overpressure
  Passive side bending to the right—overpressure
  Passive side bending to the left—overpressure
Combination passive movements
  Backward bending/side bending
  Directing a vertical force through the head into the
    cervical region
  Side bending to the left and rotation to the right with
    overpressure in a 45-degree plane of the apophyseal
    joint, reverse
Extension: fixed-point/combined end-range testing
  Passive fixed-point segmental extension—overpressure
  Passive extension/side bending/rotation away—
    overpressure
Palpation of the lateral aspect of the neck
Testing resting length: Anterior shoulder/chest

The clinician should develop a consistent palpation sequence for all patients with cervical spine problems. Using a similar routine for palpation allows for comparisons to be made between patients and gives the clinician a better sense of typical and atypical findings.

The palpation begins by identifying the C2 spinous process, the largest bony landmark and easiest spinous process to palpate. Once this landmark is identified, the clinician moves superior to the nuchal line and palpates the insertional regions of the trapezius, splenius capitis, and semispinalis capitis muscle groups. In patients with neck pain, it is common to find tenderness with palpation in these regions as well as in the suboccipital region.

The palpation continues by moving laterally from the suboccipital muscles to palpate the mastoid process. This bony prominence serves as the combined attachment of the sternocleidomastoid, longissimus capitis, and splenius capitis muscles and often is sensitive to palpation in patients with acceleration injuries of the spine or in cervical spine syndromes with prolonged and continuous muscle guarding.

Once these regions are palpated, the clinician can then return to the C2 spinous process and move one fingerbreadth laterally. This places the palpating fingers over the region of the articular pillars (inferior and superior articulating processes) of the cervical spine. The clinician should be able to palpate the raised bony ridges of the articular pillars through the cervical paraspinal muscles (Fig. 5–28). The muscularity of the patient and the degree of muscle guarding influence the ability to palpate these bony landmarks. It is common to find these bony ridges related to the apophyseal joint painful with palpation, which often is described as familiar pain. It is difficult to precisely identify the exact tissue involved because of the multiple tissue layers, but tenderness to palpation does give the clinician an idea as to the level or site of the tissue damage.

The palpation continues inferiorly, following the musculature toward the superior medial border of the scapula, which serves as the region of the levator scapulae muscle attachment. This point of the scapula often is found to be tender because it represents an area of significant muscle forces. The levator scapulae is an important muscle that works in conjunction with the other scapula muscles for stabilization of the scapula so that humeral and upper-quarter movements can take place. With the scapula fixated, it also helps to stabilize the cervical spine in the sagittal, frontal, and coronal planes. The levator scapulae can

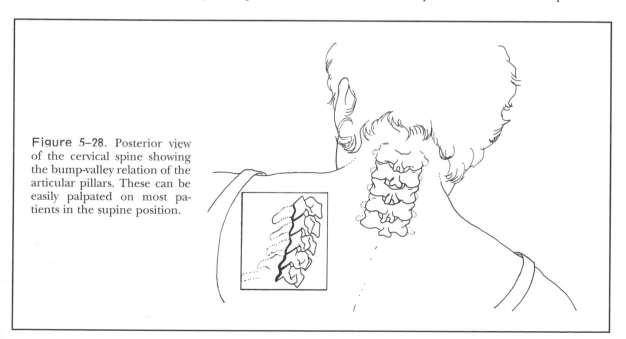

Figure 5–28. Posterior view of the cervical spine showing the bump-valley relation of the articular pillars. These can be easily palpated on most patients in the supine position.

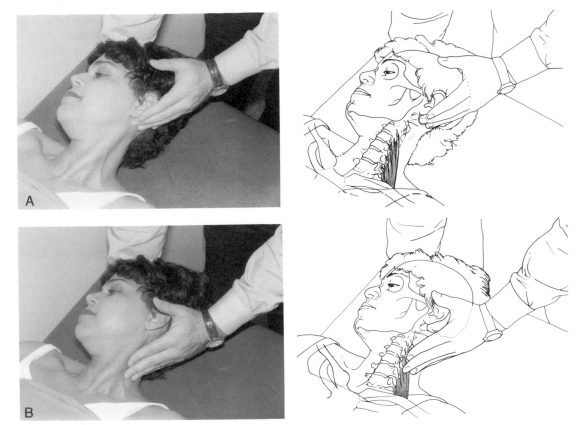

Figure 5–29. Palpation of the mastoid process (A), sternocleidomastoid, clavicle, acromio-clavicular joint, trapezius, anterior and middle scalene (B), and brachial plexus.

be injured during a rapid motion in forward bending or when overuse of the muscle is required to stabilize and counterbalance the anterior shear force of the head and neck caused by cervical lordosis or a forward-head posture.

The palpation continues over the region of the trapezius muscle out to the lateral portion of the scapula. The cervicothoracic junction often is sensitive to palpation. In this area, the trapezius muscle tissue is replaced by a fascial anchor (see Chapter 3).

Palpation continues by supporting the patient's head in the left hand and rotating the head and neck to the left. This position exposes the anterolateral aspect of the neck on the right. From this position, many structures can be appraised. The clinician can begin at the mastoid process (Fig. 5–29A) and move inferiorly along the sternoclei-

domastoid muscle to the sternoclavicular joint. The clavicle can then be followed lateral to the acromioclavicular joint. This point not only represents an articulation, but also is the lateralmost aspect of the attachment of the trapezius muscle. The clinician can follow the trapezius medial and superior to the lateral aspect of the neck.

The scalene muscle group can then be identified and palpated (Fig. 5–29B). Portions of the brachial plexus usually can be seen through the skin, especially if the neck is flexed slightly laterally by the clinician. The head is then cradled in the right hand and rotated to the right, and a similar procedure is followed on the opposite side.

Palpation of these anterolateral structures is especially important in patients with acceleration injuries of the neck. It often is necessary to gently push the visceral tube slightly lateral to assess the soft tissue over the anterior aspect of the cervical vertebral bodies. This region is covered by the longus colli muscles, which commonly are injured with a forced hyperextension motion of the neck.

Passive Range of Motion: Rotation and Side Bending with End-Range Testing

Once palpation is completed in the supine position, the clinician continues the examination by performing passive movement with overpressure testing. The patient's head is gently lifted from the table and comfortably supported in the clinician's hands. The patient is asked to relax, and a passive gentle rotation to the right is performed (Fig. 5–30A). Overpressure is applied at end range. Rotation to the left then follows with gentle overpressure at end-range rotation (Fig. 5–30B).

Passive side bending to the right (Fig. 5–31A) and left (Fig. 5–31B) with overpressure follows as the clinician attempts to evaluate not only those movements and forces that cause pain, but also the patient's willingness to allow movement. It is common for the patient to neuromuscularly guard against movements that stimulate the nociceptive receptors of injured tissue.

Combinations of movements, such as backward bending, right side bending, and right rotation, can then be used to assess the response of the cervical spine to end-range positions. Passive backward bending and side bending to the right

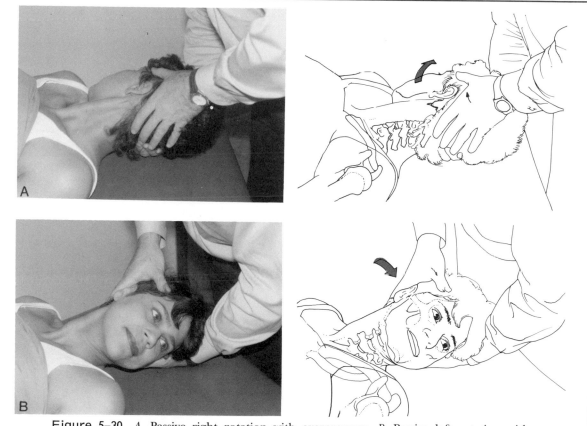

Figure 5–30. *A*, Passive right rotation with overpressure. *B*, Passive left rotation with overpressure.

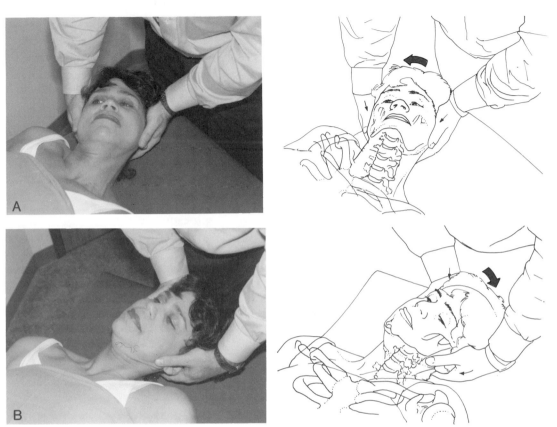

Figure 5–31. *A*, Passive side bending to the right with overpressure. *B*, Passive side bending to the left with overpressure.

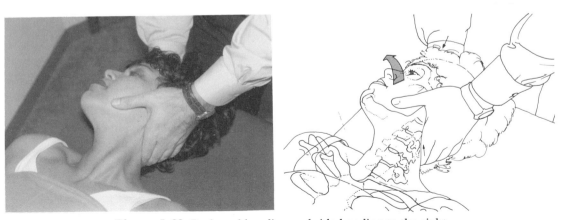

Figure 5–32. Backward bending and side bending to the right.

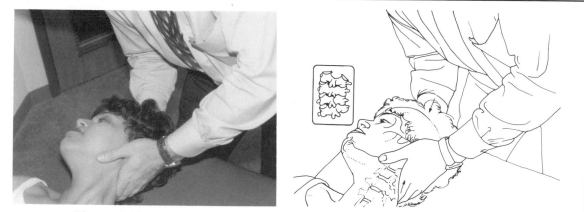

Figure 5–33. Vertical force is directed through the head into the cervical region.

is shown in Figure 5–32. A compressive force can now be generated by the clinician through the occiput and into the cervical spine (Fig. 5–33). This compression and shear force through the cervical tissues should be compared with the findings observed when the same stresses were applied in the seated examination. The same maneuver to the left is then assessed.

The patient's head and neck are then returned to the neutral position. The patient is asked first to actively backward bend in an attempt to look back toward the clinician (Fig. 5–34) and then to reverse the motion by actively flexing the neck or tucking the chin (Fig. 5–35). Overpressure can again be applied from this position.

Passive motion testing continues by combining passive left side bending and right rotation (Fig. 5–36A), followed by passive right side bending and left rotation (Fig. 5–36B). This position conflicts with the normal coupling motion of the cervical spine related to side bending and rotation (see Chapter 4). As the side-bending movement passes through midrange and the clinician begins to gently rotate the head and neck to the left, the vertebrae are directed to move against their normal mechanics.

The majority of this rotational motion occurs at the atlantoaxial joint. Once the atlantoaxial joint has reached the end range of rotation, the movement continues into the lower cervical

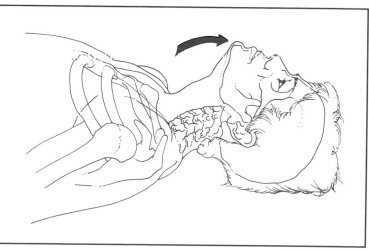

Figure 5–34. Active cervical backward bending.

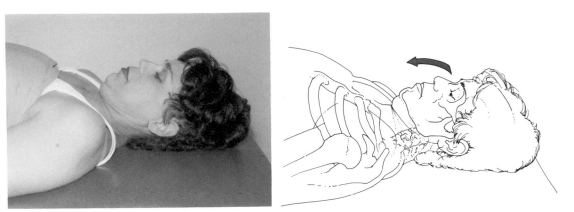

Figure 5–35. Active cervical flexion.

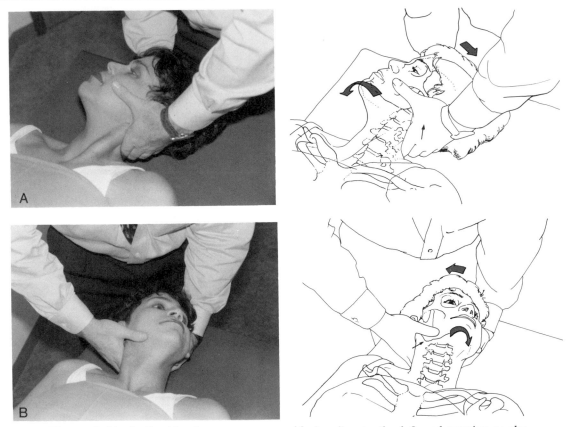

Figure 5–36. *A,* Combination movements—side bending to the left and rotation to the right with overpressure of the left hand forward and upward in a 45-degree plane of the apophyseal joint. *B,* Combination movements—side bending to the right and rotation to the left with a mobilizing hand and a stabilizing hand. Note that the movement angle of the mobilizing hand is in a 45-degree plane along the plane of the cervical apophyseal joint.

= closed pack position of facets

spine. The motion terminates at the fulcrum created by the clinician's right hand. Once the movement has reached the clinician's right hand, the force created by the clinician is anterior and superior, parallel to the joint plane. At this point, the support structures are assessed. A normal finding is a spongy end feel or an elastic feel at the end range without discomfort. A click occasionally is felt or heard, which probably indicates a change of pressure within the joint.

The clinician continues the assessment by side bending to different levels of the cervical spine and rotating the cervical spine in an opposite direction. The clinician can direct the examination forces to the upper, middle, and lower aspects of both sides of the cervical spine using hand placement as a fulcrum. The greater the range of motion in side bending, the more inferiorly in the cervical spine the forces converge. For example, the clinician's right hand can be placed in the mid cervical spine, parallel to the apophyseal joint plane. The left hand then performs the right side bending and left rotation maneuver. When end range is reached, the clinician gently lifts with the right hand as if to move the inferior articulating process anteriorly on the superior articulating process. This helps to assess the response of the cervical joints to end-range testing.

Utilizing Fixed Points for Extension Quadrant Testing

The fixed-point technique can be used to assess extension capabilities and the response to compression and shear in the cervical spine. The technique is a further refinement of extension and compression stresses that have already been introduced in the examination.

Figure 5–37 shows the technique. The clinician places the left hand in a cupped position at the mid cervical spine, with the thumb and index finger serving as the borders of the cup. With the left hand, the clinician creates an anteriorly and superiorly directed force toward the occiput about parallel to the plane of the apophyseal joints. The clinician then grasps the occiput with the right hand and gently backward bends the cervical spine over this fulcrum. The cervical spine is then returned to a neutral position by the right hand, and the cupped left hand is moved inferior along the cervical spine to assess the lower cervical segments.

By varying the direction of the force applied by way of the clinician's index finger or thumb on the cup-shaped fulcrum, the clinician can direct fairly precise extension and rotary forces to specific regions of the cervical spine. For example, backward bending and side bending to the right

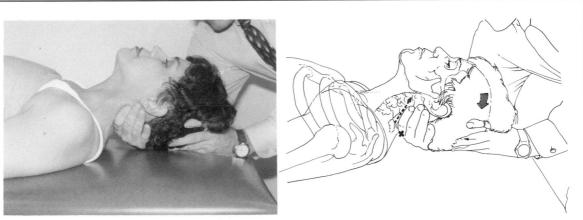

Figure 5–37. Fixed-point extension testing. The hand is in a C position at the midcervical spine. The patient's head is backward bent over the stabilizing hand. The clinician should visualize the stabilizing hand fixating the vertebrae at that site and the vertebrae above backward bending to that point.

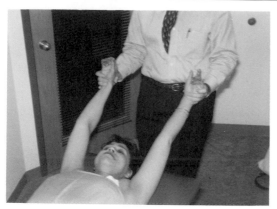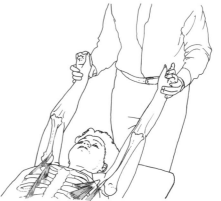

Figure 5–38. Assessment of resting length of pectoralis minor and latissimus dorsi.

with increased pressure through the index finger localizes the extension, rotation, and shear force to specific regions of the cervical spine. Not only is the quality of movement assessed, but also the ease in reproducing familiar pain, and the approximate level of the injury is better determined.

Screening the Anterior Shoulder Girdle

To complete the supine lying examination, the clinician tests the length of the scapular depressors, humeral internal rotators, and humeral adductors. The clinician grasps both of the patient's hands and brings the arms upward (Fig. 5–38). This assesses the resting length and contractile state of the pectoralis minor, pectoralis major, and latissimus dorsi muscle groups. Asymmetry, excessive arching of the spine to get the arms overhead, or the inability to reach full range of motion should be noted, and any correlation to the head and neck syndrome should be made.

Tightness is significant because scapular protraction approximates the clavicle to the first rib. This change in the position of the scapula can result in a compression of the neurovascular bundle and narrowing of the thoracic outlet (Fig. 5–39). The forward-head, round-shoulder posture results in humeral internal rotation, which narrows the subacromial space and predisposes the suprahumeral tissues to impingement.

The examination continues by passively abducting the right and left shoulders. This end

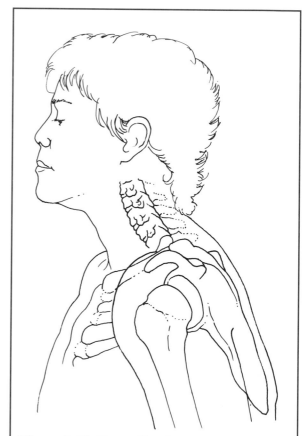

Figure 5–39. Forward-head posture, compression of the neurovascular bundle by the lateral aspect of the clavicle, and tipping of the scapula upward and forward.

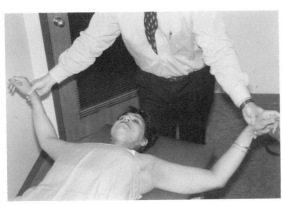
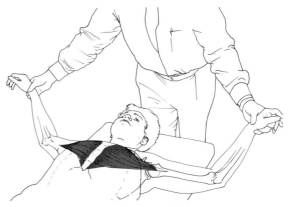

Figure 5–40. Resting length of the pectoralis major muscle and related tissues.

position assesses the resting length of the sterno-costal portion of the pectoralis major muscle and the glenohumeral joint capsule (Fig. 5–40). Tightness of the glenohumeral region is especially common in those patients who work in a prolonged sitting position.

The rounded-shoulder posture can also be furthered in women with large breasts. The anterior and inferior forces created by the weight of the breasts can result in fatigue of the thoracic and scapular musculature, which compounds the rounded-shoulder posture. Strength, power, and endurance of the scapular retractors are required to counterbalance the weight of the chest.

Assessment of the relation between the posture of the head and neck and the rest position of the shoulder girdle is important. Repositioning the head and neck so that they are in line with the shoulders is one of the main goals of the upper quarter treatment program. It must also be recognized, however, that when tightness is found, it can be due to adaptive shortening of tissues or increased efferent output to the musculature. The clinician then attempts to correlate the syndrome to the biomechanics of the tightness. In general, if the forces of the tightness increase mechanical stress to the injured region, stretching is indicated. However, if the forces of the tightness direct stresses away from the injured upper-quarter region, stretching may be contraindicated.

PRONE LYING EXAMINATION

Palpation

The patient is asked to lie prone so that the upper-quarter evaluation can be completed (Table 5–5). A pillow is placed beneath the chest so that the patient's forehead can either rest on the plinth or fit securely into an opening in the plinth (Fig. 5–41). On a variety of plinths, a section can be removed to allow freedom to breathe with the cervical spine in the neutral position. This adaptation of the treatment table permits comfortable positioning, which augments the prone lying examination and certain treatment procedures. If this feature is not available, the clinician should be aware that a rotated cervical spine creates excessive forces to the cervical spine and should be avoided.

Palpation in the prone position can begin at the occiput (nuchal line) and proceed inferiorly

Table 5–5. Prone Lying Examination
Palpation: Occiput to C2 spinous process (suboccipitals) to acromion to scapula to mid thoracic spine up spinous processes to cervical spine. Should correlate with supine findings. This position for palpation is mainly needed for those areas that cannot be palpated in the supine position
Correlation of findings to the radiograph: View radiographs if available.

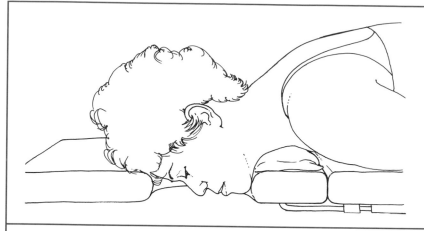

Figure 5–41. Positioning of the patient using a removable portion of the treatment table.

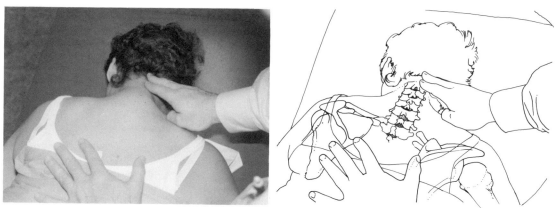

Figure 5–42. Palpation of the suboccipital region—C2 spinous process.

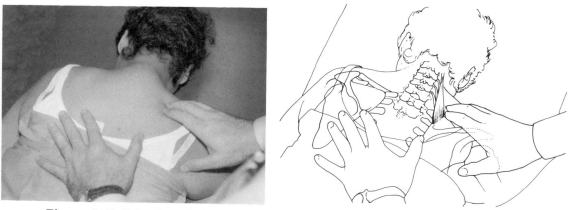

Figure 5–43. Palpation of the superior medial border of the right scapula (trapezius–levator scapulae).

to identify the C2 spinous process (Fig. 5–42). From this starting point, the remaining soft tissues of the posterior aspect of the cervical spine and scapula can then be palpated (Fig. 5–43).

From this position, the thoracic and scapular regions should be palpated. The findings during palpation in this position should closely correlate with those established in the supine position. Areas of increased tissue tension and muscle guarding and the response to pressure over the soft tissue should be assessed.

Gentle posteroanterior pressures can also be placed over the segments of the cervical and upper thoracic spine, either directly over the spinous processes or over the region of the articular pillars. This often is uncomfortable to patients, and care must be taken when using this assessment. With this palpation, the clinician is assessing the response of the patient to anterior shear stresses and joint compression of the cervical spine.

Posterior-to-anterior pressures can also be applied over the upper ribs from this position. This force causes a traction (separation) force at the costotransverse joints and should be considered a potential source of pain, especially if the person complains of pain with deep inspiration or during heavy exertion.

This concludes the examination of the upper quarter of the patient with neck pain. The last aspect of the assessment is to view the results of the diagnostic tests, particularly the radiographs.

CORRELATION OF FINDINGS TO THE RADIOGRAPH OR IMAGING STUDY

The last judgment during the functional assessment is to correlate the findings of the physical examination with the radiographic or imaging

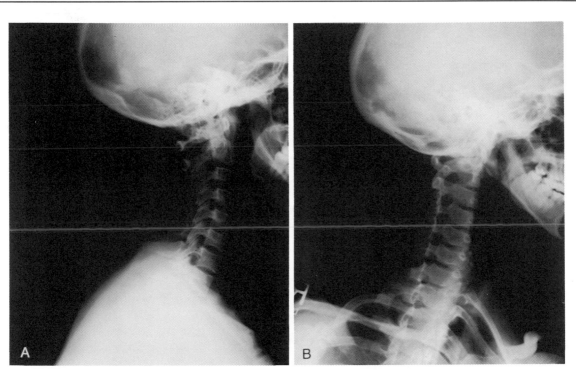

Figure 5–44. Radiograph showing changes in the shape of the vertebral bodies of the cervical spine. *A,* Lateral view; *B,* oblique view.

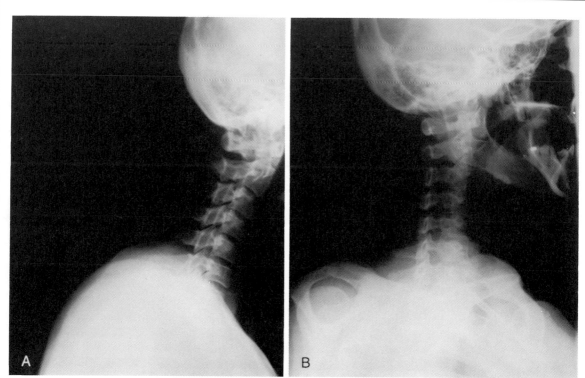

Figure 5–45. Radiographs showing the sclerosis of the apophyseal joint of the cervical spine.

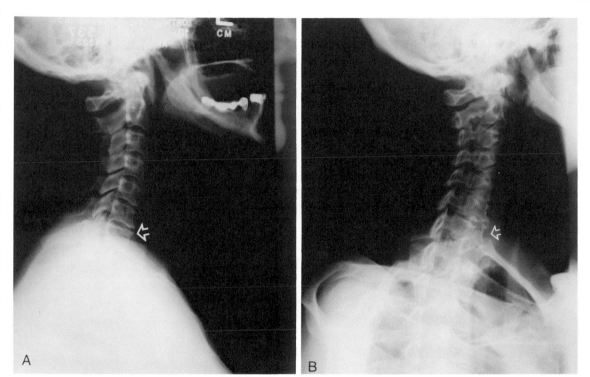

Figure 5–46. Radiographs showing significant cervical disc height changes. The arrows indicate degenerative disc, causing a narrowed disc space. Consider the increased load at the apophyseal joint and the altered size and mechanics of the neuroforamen.

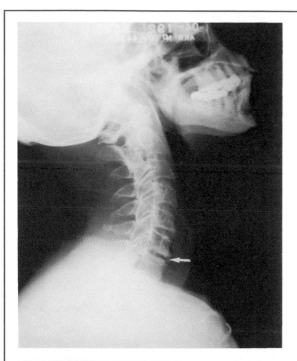

Figure 5–47. Extension (backward bending) x-ray showing decreased motion at the C6,C7 region and showing very little motion at that segment. Note the sclerosis between the C6,C7 disc space.

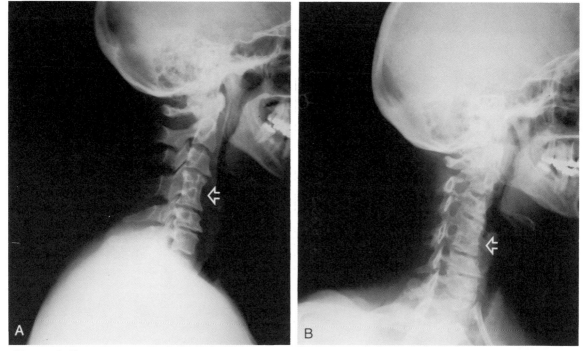

Figure 5–48. *A*, Lateral view revealing fusion of C4,C5 vertebra. Note the significant change in the cervical lordosis and recognize the adaptations that must take place to maintain that position. *B*, Oblique view showing the same interbody fusion at C4,C5. The neuroforamen are open.

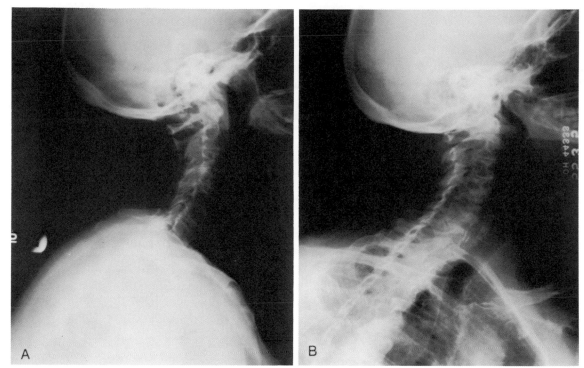

Figure 5–49. *A,* Lateral view. Significant changes in bone mass and degeneration of the cervical spine. *B,* Oblique view. Note significant narrowing of the vertebral foramen at the low lumbar vertebral segments.

assessment, if one is available. Based on the assessment, the clinician should be able to reasonably predict the imaging findings by the results of pain pattern, pain location, length of time the patient has had pain, passive and active mobility testing, and palpation.

Reviewing the radiographic findings helps to correlate various aspects of this physical assessment. Although there may not be a significant relation between the radiographic findings and the painful location, viewing the radiograph after completing the physical assessment often provides the clinician with a confirmation of the state of the degenerative process.[1] Figure 5–44 shows normal lateral and oblique radiographs. Figures 5–45 through 5–49 are examples of common findings on lateral and oblique views. Structural changes represent breakdown of the specialized connective tissues and the body's response to excessive forces, degeneration, and disease. Reduction of the cervical lordosis or any type of frontal

plane deviation is probably a result of protective muscle guarding and should be interpreted cautiously.

DIFFERENTIAL DIAGNOSIS

For the purpose of this text, three differential diagnoses are outlined regarding disorders of the neck. Other differential diagnosis exist[30] but are not commonly confirmed.

The first category of differential diagnosis is inflammatory disease, particularly rheumatoid arthritis. Patients with rheumatoid arthritis typically have three common patterns of cervical involvement: atlantoaxial subluxation, cranial settling or occipitoatlanto impaction syndrome, and subaxial subluxation. Cervical instability can be a complication of rheumatoid arthritis due to these patterns of involvement. In addition, the weakening of the connective tissue caused by the disease process leaves the cervical spine vulnerable to instability. The clinician needs to be aware of these possible complications and use caution in the evaluation and treatment of the neck.

The second differential diagnosis that a clinician should be aware of is neoplastic conditions. Primary cervical neoplasms are rare, but the spine is a common site for metastases from primary sites such as the prostate gland and lungs in men and the breasts in women, followed by metastases from tumors in the gastrointestinal tract and the kidneys. The spine can also be a secondary site for complications from lymphomas and myelomas. Neck pain caused by a neoplasm is localized and unrelenting and more intense at night, at rest, and during times of inactivity.

The third differential diagnosis is infections of the neck. These are most common in children, elderly people, and medically compromised patients. Clinical findings include extreme guarding, limitation of motion, and exquisite tenderness. These patients also may present with other signs of infections, such as fever, and other system dysfunction and illness.

WORKING ASSESSMENT

Once the differential diagnoses have been ruled out, a compilation of the findings from the history and the examination provides the information required to establish a logical treatment plan. This plan is designed to effectively reach realistic short- and long-term goals. To be able to design reachable short-term goals, the following information must be determined from the assessment process:

1. Pathomechanics that reproduce the familiar pain
2. Classification category of the patient's syndrome
3. Level of understanding or knowledge the patient exhibits regarding his or her condition

The following explanation defines these parameters as the basis for the development of a treatment plan that can meet the objectives of the patient and the clinician.

Pathomechanics of Familiar Pain: Pathomechanical Diagnosis

The pathomechanical diagnosis represents the movements, positions, and forces that reproduce the familiar symptoms. For example, the conclusion might be that backward bending and side bending to the right in the cervical spine increase familiar pain on the right or that forward bending and side bending to the left increase pain on the left. Using such terminology helps to standardize communication between clinicians.

Even though the pathomechanical diagnosis provides a foundation for patient education and treatment, it does not provide a complete description of the syndrome. Additional information is provided by using terminology that accurately describes the site of the patient's complaint. The Quebec Task Force studied the dilemma of standardizing the diagnosis for low back pain and recognized the inability to name the specific tissues that cause the pain.[23] As a result of this dilemma, the task force suggested a more realistic diagnostic classification scheme for activity-related spinal disorders. The diagnoses relevant to physical therapy management of mechanical low back disorders are listed in Table 5–6.[8]

Table 5–6. Quebec Task Force Categories for Low Back Pain

Low back pain without radiation
Low back pain with referral proximal
Low back pain with referral distal
Low back pain with referral with neurological signs
Leg pain worse than back pain
Post surgery less than 6 months
Post surgery greater than 6 months
Spinal stenosis
Chronic low back pain syndrome

Table 5–7. Diagnostic Classification for Mechanical Neck Pain

Neck pain without radiation
Neck pain with referral proximally
Neck pain with referral distally
Arm pain worse than neck pain
Neck pain with radiation with neurological signs
Post surgery less than 6 months
Post surgery greater than 6 months
Chronic pain syndrome

The diagnostic classification scheme for the neck can be adapted from this model (Table 5–7). Describing the syndrome in these terms affords greater reliability when discussing the syndrome with other clinicians. Such a description also allows for outcome measures to be more closely linked to a standard diagnostic scheme. Only through this type of standardization can effective treatment outcomes be measured.

To assess the usefulness of this diagnostic system, a multiuser group needs to be established with clear criteria that will permit the study of such a system. The use of this standard communication system will empower the clinician to better define and narrow the neck pain patient population. Once this is accomplished, treatment outcome data can be collected per category. Through such a system, research to define the efficacy of treatment can be developed and implemented.

Classification of Activity-Related Spinal Disorders

Thus far, we have classified the disorder by pathomechanics and pain location. The last step is to classify the patient symptom by pain pattern. This aspect of classification should be simple enough to direct a rational application of treatment techniques. It is important to develop a classification system that is complete enough to include most patients, yet simple and logical enough so that it can be used by many clinicians as a basis for discussion and research.

With this understanding, a classification that can be of use is one that places the patient in one of three categories: acute injury, reinjury or exacerbation of previous injury, or chronic pain syndrome.

In a patient with acute injury, the response to the applied stresses of the examination is proportional to the time and physical trauma of the injury or the onset of pain. The reinjury or exacerbation of previous injury classification includes patients with recurrent episodes of the same symptoms. Their explanation of each episode is relatively consistent, yet the intensity, frequency, and duration of the symptom pattern can alter. Depending on the elapsed time from the original onset of pain, the parameters of the pain pattern usually increase in duration and intensity. For example, if the patient had the original onset of pain 7 years ago and has experienced five episodes of the same syndrome, the changes that accompany age and functional adaptations often are responsible for increases in the pain pattern.

The third classification is the patient with chronic pain syndrome. To properly understand this category of patients, chronic pain syndrome needs to be defined. Most definitions include a time from onset of pain in months or years. The chronicity of the syndrome is not solely determined by the the time frame, however. In this definition of chronic pain syndrome, the patient has adopted illness behavior, hopelessness, anguish, discouragement, emotional upheaval, and disability.[28] Recognition of this influence of pain on behavior is essential because focusing treatment on modulating pain with this category of patients without attention to the psychosocial factors that influence the pain often is frustrating for both the clinician and the patient. Instead, the treatment focus should be on restoration of function, especially those changes that can be objectively measured and demonstrated to the patient.

Level of Understanding or Knowledge of the Condition

Educating the patient with respect to the results of the assessment and defining the role of the patient and the clinician in the treatment process are critical to the successful outcome of the management program. The patient must assume major responsibility for the treatment outcome. At first, the patient may not recognize the extent of the injury or the healing parameters required for functional recovery. The patient also does not have an understanding of the pain pattern.

Placing the problem in the proper perspective is essential for successful treatment outcome. Each patient can be placed along a continuum from one who is extremely active and continues to reinjure himself but refuses to take the time to properly address the problem to one who considers his condition to be the most devastating occurrence that has ever transpired. Each of these extremes and all points along the continuum represent different challenges for the clinician. For the patient who essentially is in denial and refuses to alter his or her activity, the clinician must focus on education so that the patient can identify the reasons why modification of activity and attention to the condition are warranted. At the other end of the continuum is the patient with many psychosocial factors that influence the painful syndrome. The clinician must make a judgment as to what course of action is best indicated for each patient and the factors that influence the painful syndrome. The clinician's goal should be to treat the patient as little as possible and to assist the patient to become effective in self-management.

SUMMARY

There are many ways to assess the patient with mechanical neck pain. The emphasis in this chapter is an assessment of the pathomechanics of injury and the relation of this information to an understanding of the injury as well as inflammatory and degenerative processes. In addition, the influence of environmental and personal stressors needs to be considered in the evaluation of these patients.

This assessment process does not use the assessment of segmental mobility for the purposes of quantifying motion because there is no known correlate between mobility findings and the actual syndrome, except in the case of instability of the spine. Instead, segmental motion is assessed for the purpose of reproducing the patient's pain and gaining a clearer understanding of the approximate level of the cervical spine that might be involved.

A standardized method of communication regarding diagnosis is essential if meaningful outcome studies are to be performed. For this reason, three aspects of diagnosis are presented: the pathomechanics that reproduce familiar pain, the precise location of the pain pattern, and a description of the pain pattern.

After the findings from the assessment process have been compiled, organized, and integrated, a treatment plan can be developed and implemented.

REFERENCES

1. Boden SD, McCowin PR, Davis DO, et al: Abnormal magnetic resonance scans of the cervical spine in asymptomatic subjects. J Bone Joint Surg [Am] 72:1178–1184, 1990.
2. Bogduk N, Marsland A: The cervical apophyseal joints as a source of pain. Spine 13:610–617, 1988.
3. Bosomoff HL, Fishbain D, Rosomoff RS: Chronic cervical pain: Radiculopathy or brachialgia. Spine 17:S362–S366, 1992.
4. Buchwald D, Cheney PR, Peterson DL, et al: A chronic illness characterized by fatigue, neurologic and immunologic disorders, and active human herpes virus type 6 infection. Ann Intern Med 116:103–112, 1992.
5. Butler DS. Mobilisation of the Nervous System. Melbourne, Churchill Livingstone, 1991.
6. Chan CW, Golman S, Illstrup DM, et al: The pain drawing and Waddell's nonorganic physical signs in chronic low back pain. Spine 18:1717–1722, 1993.
7. Cyriax J: Textbook of Orthopedic Medicine. Vol. 1. London, Bailliere-Tindall, 1978.
8. DeRosa CP, Porterfield JA: A physical therapy model for the treatment of low back pain. Phys Ther 72:261–269, 1992.
9. Fan PT, Blanton ME: Clinical features and diagnosis of fibromyalgia. J Musculoskel Med 9:24–42, 1992.
10. Friberg O: Clinical symptoms and biomechanics of lumbar spine and hip joint. Spine 6:643–651, 1983.
11. Gracovetsky S, Farfan HF, Helleur C: The abdominal mechanism. Spine 10:317, 1985.
12. Greenfield S, Fitzcharles MA, Esdaile JM: Reactive fibromyalgia syndrome. Arthritis Rheum 35:678–681, 1992.
13. Guyten AC: Physics of blood, blood flow, and pressure: Hemodynamics. In Textbook of Medical Physiology. Philadelphia, WB Saunders, 1981, pp 208–217.
14. Guyten AC: The lymphatic system, interstitial dynamics, edema, and pulmonary fluids. In Textbook of Medical Physiology. Philadelphia, WB Saunders, 1981, pp 370–380.
15. Hudson JI, Goldenberg DL, Pope HG, et al: Comorbidity of fibromyalgia with medical and psychiatric disorders. Am J Med 92:363–367, 1992.
16. Hurley JV: The sequence of events. In Vane JR, Ferreira SH (eds): Inflammation. Handbook of Experimental Pharmacology. Vol. 50/I. New York, Springer-Verlag, 1978, Ch 2.
17. Kendall FP, McCreary EK: Muscles Testing and Function. Baltimore, Williams & Wilkins, 1993.
18. Magee DJ: Orthopaedic Physical Assessment. Philadelphia, WB Saunders, 1987.
19. Maitland GD: Vertebral Manipulation. 5th ed. London, Butterworths, 1986, p 182.
20. May KP, West SG, Baker MR, Everett DW: Sleep apnea in male patients with fibromyalgia syndrome. Am J Med 94:505–507, 1993.
21. Neeck G, Riedel W: Thyroid function in patients with fibromyalgia syndrome. J Rheumatol 19:1120–1122, 1992.
22. Porterfield JA, DeRosa CP: Mechanical Low Back Pain:

Perspectives in Functional Anatomy. Philadelphia, WB Saunders, 1991.

23. Report of the Quebec Task Force: Scientific approach to the assessment and management of activity-related spinal disorders. Spine 12:S-16, 1987.

24. Rocabado M, Iglarsh ZA: Musculoskeletal Approach to Maxillofacial Pain. Philadelphia, JB Lippincott, 1991.

25. Russell IJ, Michalek JE, Vipraio GA, et al: Platelet 3H-imipramine uptake receptor density and serum serotonin levels in patients with fibromyalgia/fibrositis syndrome. J Rheumatol 19:104–109, 1992.

26. Simms RW, Zerbini CA, Ferrante N, et al: Fibromyalgia syndrome in patients infected with human immunodeficiency virus. Am J Med 92:368–374, 1992.

27. Symthe H: Links between fibromyalgia and myofascial pain syndrome (editorial). J Rheumatol 19:842–843, 1992.

28. Waddell G, McCullouch JA: Nonorganic physical signs in low back pain. Spine 5:117–125, 1980.

29. Waddell G: A new clinical model for the treatment of low back pain. Spine 12:632–644, 1987.

30. Weisel SW, Feffer HL, Rothman RH: Non-mechanical causes of neck pain. In Neck Pain. Charlottesville, VA, Michie Co, 1986, pp 87–246.

31. Wolt CJ: Generation of acute pain: Central mechanisms. Br Med Bull 47:523–533, 1991.

32. Wolfe F, Smythe HA, Yunus MB, et al: The American College of Rheumatology: Criteria for the classification of fibromyalgia: Report of the Multicenter Criteria Committee. Arthritis Rheum 33:160–172, 1990.

33. Woo SL-Y, Buckwalter JA: Injury and Repair of the Musculoskeletal Soft Tissues. Park Ridge, IL, American Academy of Orthopedic Surgeons, 1988.

34. Youlten LJF: Inflammatory mediators and vascular events. In Vane JR, Ferreira SH (eds): Inflammation. Handbook of Experimental Pharmacology. Vol. 50/I. New York, Springer-Verlag, 1978, pp 571–586.

35. Yunus MB: Towards a model of pathophysiology of fibromyalgia: Aberrant central pain mechanisms with peripheral modulation (editorial). J Rheumatol 19:846–850, 1992.

CHAPTER 6

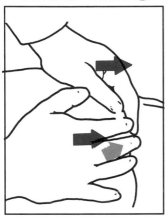

TREATMENT OF MECHANICAL NECK DISORDERS

Economic changes have necessitated a redirection of management strategies for spinal disorders. In the past, a wide array of treatment techniques, ranging from high-velocity manipulation to palliative heat and massage, were available to the clinician; the emphasis on cost-effectiveness and efficiency has resulted in developing treatment approaches aimed at maximizing the reactivation of the patient and developing the skills required for self-management. In addition, it is apparent that the patient must assume an active role in attaining a successful outcome.

The scope of this chapter is not to debate the effectiveness of the techniques involved in treating neck disorders, but to integrate assessment findings into a treatment plan based on the science of soft tissue healing and age-related changes in spinal tissues. The concepts are based on a pragmatic educational process that significantly involves the patient in self-care. Correlating assessment findings to a treatment plan and communicating this information to the patient are crucial to a successful outcome. The patient must become aware of the subtle changes in intensity, frequency, and duration of the syndrome to participate in self-management. This increased awareness should also be communicated to the clinician to determine the future direction of treatment.

The clinician and patient must be able to communicate with each other. The success of the treatment process depends on the clinician's ability to explain the neuromuscular and musculoskeletal science to the patient in a logical, understandable manner. Greater patient understanding leads to reduced anxiety and increases the patient's willingness to participate in the process.

Setting and attaining realistic short-term goals is the key to gaining patient confidence. After the short-term goals are accomplished, realistic long-term goals are set. A program should be developed that will satisfy a patient's needs, rather than the clinician's perception of a patient's needs. The most efficient management of patients with spinal disorders occurs when the clinician can integrate the science of soft tissue healing, the psychosocial influences on the syndrome, and the patients' willingness to accept responsibility for their condition. Whether the

173

pain arises from tendon, ligament, bone, or nerve is not the key issue. Rather, the focus should be the patient's ability to successfully integrate the knowledge gained from the rehabilitation process into activities of daily living. An active, relatively painless life-style is the goal. The patient's role is to actively participate in the treatment process by integrating information and modifying activities with respect to the pain pattern. The clinician's role is to assist the patient in determining the parameters of the pain pattern and in recognizing the parameters that exacerbate the symptoms. The clinician is the director and instructor of the treatment process, and the patient is the student, analyst, and assistant.

In the practice of modern physical medicine, the question arises, To what extent should we treat patients who do not want to take responsibility and be held accountable for their syndromes? We should not prematurely discontinue those who have difficulty grasping the concepts because people learn and integrate information at different levels and at varying speeds. All the clinician can ask of the patient is a concerted effort and the motivation to improve. Those in a small subset of the patient population who do not want to help themselves represent those who do not respond favorably to treatment and who contribute disproportionately to the rising cost of treating spinal disorders. If the patient does not possess the necessary mental and emotional capacity or other extraneous circumstances hamper the patient's ability to control his or her actions, then appropriate referral is indicated. Consistent passive treatment that lacks a high level of communication is certainly not indicated. The successful clinician can rapidly and accurately identify the patient's willingness and ability to take control of the condition.

The following explanation of the treatment process begins with the intent of treatment, followed by the development of the objectives of treatment, and concludes with an introduction of a treatment model.

TREATMENT STRATEGY

The intent of treatment has seven distinct components. They are as follows:

1. Educate the patient.
2. Maximize the healing potential.
3. Establish short- and long-term goals.
4. Restore the anatomical relation between injured and noninjured tissues.
5. Maintain the normal function of the noninjured tissue.
6. Avoid placing excessive strain on the injured area.
7. Optimize cost-effectiveness by assisting the patient in becoming an educated health care consumer.

These goals are accomplished by designing an individualized treatment strategy based on a logical explanation of the assessment findings and the establishment of realistic treatment goals endorsed by the patient. The overall intention is to see the patient as few times as possible to reach the desired goal of patient control.

Educating the Patient: Explanation of Assessment Findings and Implementation of Treatment Plan

Immediately after assessment of the upper quarter, the clinician should begin a discussion of the findings and conclusions. This educational process is an important first step of the treatment program. Education provides the patient with an understanding of the logic behind the design of the treatment program. Perhaps more important, it promotes the idea that the patient and the clinician must work together in determining the direction and progression of care. Both need to be cognizant of the physical and perceptual changes that occur as a result of treatment.

This information can be constructively presented so that the patient can make use of the knowledge in the decision-making processes during rehabilitation. It is the clinician's challenge to develop the patient's knowledge base so that this information can be presented effectively. Understanding the basic science is crucial for the patient who wants to maximize treatment results and overall health. This learning represents the first and most important step toward directing responsibility for treatment outcome from the medical practitioner to the patient. Knowledge empowers the patient to make the kinds of necessary decisions during the activities of daily liv-

Table 6–1. Outline of the Discussion Following the Assessment

I. Structure of the neck and shoulder complex
  A. Cervical segment anatomy and function
    1. Intervertebral disc
      a. Annulus
      b Nucleus
      c. Normal function
      d. Degeneration process
      e. Herniation
    2. Cervical apophyseal joint
      a. Articular cartilage
      b. Normal function
      c. Degeneration (Overuse syndrome)
      d. Mid/end range weight bearing
  B. Injury cycle (Figure 6–2)
      a. Injury causes pain;
      b. Pain causes spasm and fatigue
      c. Spasm causes
        1. Decreased blood flow
        2. Congestion of fluid (Figure 6–3)
        3. Increased pressure causes
          a. hypoxia
          b. biochemical exchange
            1. chemical irritation
              (PAIN)
      d. Fatigue causes
        1. Decreased protection and increased
          mechanical stresses which cause increased
          (PAIN)
        2. Pain decreases physical activity
  C. Disrupting the injury cycle
      a. Altered by modalities to enhance blood flow
        and minimize fluid congestion
  D. Establishing the short term and long term goals
      a. Pain generated
      b. Function generated to be detailed later

vertebral body, intervertebral disc, apophyseal joint, nerve root, neuroforamen, and spinal canal. The discussion continues by describing the structure and function of the annulus fibrosis and nucleus pulposus of the intervertebral disc. This includes an explanation of the contributions the annulus and nucleus make in the stabilization of the cervical spine. Depending on the diagnosis and assessment findings, the discussion can progress into an explanation of age-related changes, the degenerative process, or the sequence of disc pathology. It is also important to describe conditions related to encroachment at the neuroforamen or spinal canal. This is especially relevant because of the high incidence of cervical spondylosis.

Following the discussion of the cervical spine, a brief overview of the musculature can be provided. Muscles can be described as motors that can be injured or assume increased states of contraction as a response to injury or emotional stress that generate the forces of gravity and movement into and through the skeletal tissues.

Many patients have misconceptions about the structure and function of the articular cartilage. Articular cartilage is shown and the results of overload or overuse described in Figure 6–1. Using the metacarpophalangeal joints of the patient's hand as an example of the concept of midrange and end range and then relating this example to the actions of the apophyseal joints of the neck is quite effective. By illustrating weight bearing of the normal segment versus that of the degenerative segment, the patient can begin to better understand the anatomical and physiological changes associated with injury and segment degeneration and at the same time begin to realize how the clinician thinks.

A radiograph of the patient's cervical spine can supplement the educational process. It significantly adds to the quality and effectiveness of the discussion because it allows the patient to visualize the age-related changes of the cervical spine. Positive treatment outcomes are directly related to the quality of patient-clinician interaction.

The clinician should refrain from using terms such as rupture, herniation, and degeneration because the patient's interpretation may be markedly different from what is intended by the clinician. These terms connote explosiveness, which most often is interpreted by the patient as leading

ing that are crucial for successful long-term management of an upper-quarter condition. Painless, active function should be at the forefront of patient goals.

Tools that can assist in the educational process include an anatomical model of the upper quarter, appropriate anatomical illustrations, and tools for writing and drawing. Table 6–1 provides a suggested discussion outline the clinician can follow with the patient. After this discussion, a treatment plan and home program can be proposed.

It is most useful to begin the discussion of the upper quarter by defining the vertebral segment of the cervical spine. The relevant anatomy of the segment includes the relationships between the

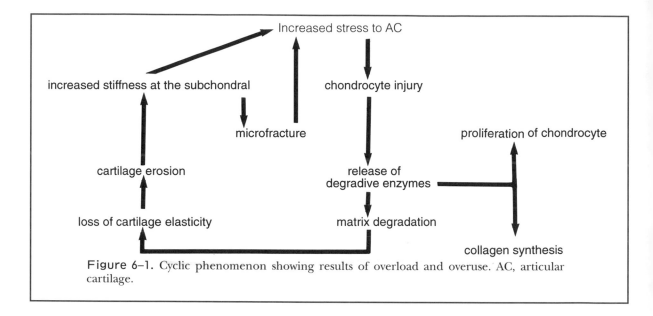

Figure 6–1. Cyclic phenomenon showing results of overload and overuse. AC, articular cartilage.

to dismal treatment outcomes. This impression may lead to the conversion of simple neck pain into an exaggerated unmanageable pain syndrome.

Maximizing the Healing Potential

The second intent of treatment of the musculoskeletal tissues is to create an optimal tissue environment that best uses the body's potential for functional repair. The body has an efficient healing mechanism for these tissues. However, depending on a person's health and age, the time frames vary (Table 6–2).[4, 8, 12] Tissues that stabilize the movable segment, such as ligaments, tendons, and fascia, take up to 12 weeks to heal, barring a significant exacerbation in the process.

The healing process of musculoskeletal tissue

Table 6–2. Healing Phases of the Neuromusculoskeletal System			
	Reaction Phase *Inflammatory Reaction*	**Regeneration Phase** *Repair and Healing*	**Remodeling Phase** *Maturation and Remodeling*
Physiological Activities:	Vascular changes	Removal of noxious stimuli	Maturation of connective tissue
	Exudation of cells and chemicals	Growth of capillary beds into area	Contracture of scar tissue
	Clot formation	Collagen formation	Remodeling of scar
	Phagocytosis, neutralization of irritants	Granulation tissue	Collagen aligns to stress
	Early fibroblastic activity	Very fragile, easily injured tissue	
Clinical Signs:	Inflammation	Decreasing inflammation	Absence of inflammation
	Pain before tissue resistance	Pain synchronous with tissue resistance	Pain after tissue resistance
Time Frame:	Up to 74 hours	48 hours up to 6 weeks	3 weeks to 12 months

Note the extended time required for healing of collagenous structures. There are a variety of treatment methods that are effective in temporarily desensitizing the tissues, thereby decreasing pain. However, a decrease in pain should not be the measure of healing. The clinician must remain aware of the time required for functional healing so that proper decisions can be made regarding return to activity (work). In the industrial setting, education to the management regarding this reality significantly improves the likelihood for successful return to work. The goal of the return to work (activity) is gradual progressive loading without reexacerbation of the original injury.

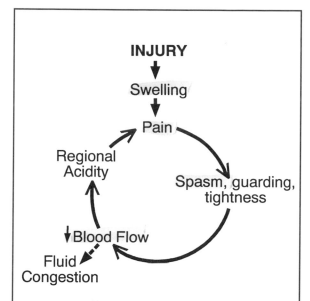

INJURY

Swelling

Pain

Regional
Acidity

Spasm, guarding,
tightness

↓Blood Flow

Fluid
Congestion

Figure 6–2. Injury cycle. Injury causes swelling and pain. Pain results in spasm or protective guarding. This sustained contraction alters fluid dynamics as a result of decreased blood flow, causing congestion of fluid. Fluid congestion increases pressure and slows the biochemical exchange necessary for increased metabolism of repair. Fluid congestion also causes peripheral hypoxia. The absence of oxygen in the tissue creates pH changes or a biochemical imbalance within the environment, which results in further chemical irritation to the afferent chemoreceptor and increases pain.

is a series of chemical events and physical results that takes on a cyclic arrangement called the injury cycle (Fig. 6–2). This cycle is a condensed version of the injury-degeneration cycle introduced in Chapter 5. The cycle is simplified for explanation to the patient. The outline in Table 6–1 indicates the point at which the injury cycle typically is discussed. Because not all patients recall an injury at the beginning of an upper-quarter syndrome, the definition of an injury can be expanded to include a rapid or gradual onset of symptoms. Patients who have early degenerative changes commonly recall trauma to the head and neck early in their lives. For example, a 45-year-

old patient with a degenerative cervical segment should be asked, "Have you ever experienced a blow to the head or any other traumatic event to the head and neck?" Although this information usually is not alluded to during the initial portion of the history, it can provide a rationale for early degeneration. Specialized connective tissues, such as articular cartilage of the apophyseal joints or the cervical intervertebral discs, break down by a gradual progressive overload or a rapid impact. Both processes take considerable time to become symptomatic.

The healing environment can be maximized when the patient understands the concepts of fluid congestion and stasis and how blood flow and lymph drainage are altered with musculoskeletal injury. The most efficient way to minimize stasis is through active movement. Armed with this information, the patient now understands why controlled active movement is necessary for the healing process.

It should be explained to the patient that inflammation is a natural occurrence after injury that needs to be controlled through proper decision-making (balance between rest and activity) and early nondestructive movement (therapeutic exercise). The resolution of the problem appears to be prompt intervention and a program designed to restore normal fluid dynamics.

The healing environment can be optimized only if stasis is minimized. The results of fluid stasis include increased accumulation of tissue byproducts and an altered chemical milieu (Fig. 6–3). This chemical environment sensitizes the afferent nerve terminals surrounding the injured tissues. The exudate has been referred to as "sensitizing soup."[11] Prompt intervention is important because this "soup" maintains a fluid-like consistency for about 3 to 4 days that can be easily managed. If, however, the injury is not properly managed, the "soup" begins to organize and becomes gel-like, which makes it difficult to evacuate. The presentation continues by two lines drawn through the injury cycle, signifying that the short-term goal of treatment is to interrupt this physiological cycle (Fig. 6–4). Altering the cycle is accomplished by using the modalities, manual techniques, or activities that enhance fluid movement. Modalities and their use are further explained in the first objective of treatment: Pain modulation or promotion of analgesia.

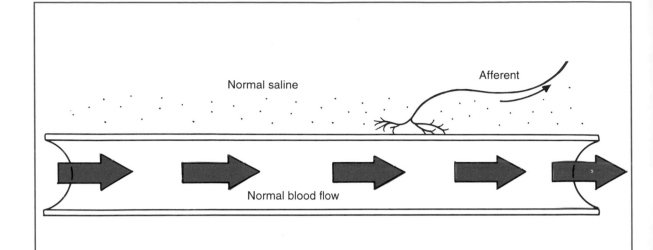

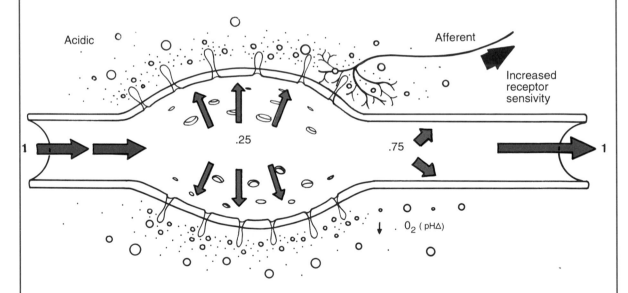

Figure 6–3. Fluid congestion phenomenon. The clinician can draw two parallel lines that signify a blood vessel. Arrows can be placed within those lines depicting the flow of fluid, either blood or extracellular fluid (lymph). Patients can relate to the thought that before the onset of symptom (injury), the fluid movement was uninhibited. The clinician can continue by showing the changes in the bottom drawing, which represent the result of the inflammatory process. The blood flow enters the injured region, slows, and then exits. In this congested area, there is an increase in pressure. The tissues at the periphery of that pressure become deprived of oxygen, resulting in increased production and accumulation of metabolites and altered pH. There is now an acidic medium or "sensitizing soup."[11] This results in neural hypersensitivity, which causes the cycle to continue.[10]

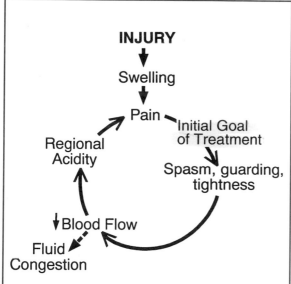

INJURY

Swelling

Pain — Initial Goal of Treatment

Regional Acidity

Spasm, guarding, tightness

↓Blood Flow

Fluid Congestion

Figure 6–4. Disruption of the injury cycle, signifying the short-term goal of the initial aspect of the treatment process. This cycle is broken by the use of thermal, electrical, manual, and medical modalities.

Establishing Short- and Long-Term Goals

A practical way to establish short- and long-term goals is to relate back to the graphs. The following is an example of the discussion regarding setting the short-term goal. Most patients who enter an outpatient clinic with upper-quarter complaints share the same immediate goals: decrease the pain and improve the function. The clinician can refer to the graphs and demonstrate to the patient that the goal is to lessen the intensity of the syndrome. Short-term goals can be explained from the graph of the daily behavior of pain. Morning stiffness, which is present in many patients with age-related changes, should decrease as the clinician and patient realize successes from initial management strategies.

Long-term goals become clearer as painless function increases. Most patients can express their long-term goals at the onset of treatment, but as changes in function occur as a result of treatment, long-term goals can be reestablished. The long-term goal often is not accomplished within the supervised medical treatment plan. Successful fulfillment of long-term goals undoubtedly consists of adopting health habits that best afford the patient relief and control. The detail of the health habits should be the basis for the home program.

Educational Additions with Cases That Involve Many Variables

After taking the patient's history, the clinician should have a relatively clear understanding as to the complexity of the syndrome. For example, if the patient has an understandable injury with no prior pain, a logically progressing functional assessment, a high rating on the activity scale, and a low rating on the stress scale, then the clinician can conclude that the syndrome has a much greater chance for resolution.

Conversely, if the patient has a difficult time organizing his or her thoughts and the clinician learns to appreciate that the upper-quarter syndrome is compounded by stressors in the patient's life, the success of the treatment process depends on the patient's ability to recognize the interrelationships of the many variables that perpetuate the syndrome.

The patient in this category is one who has a low rating on the activity scale and a high rating on the stress scale. If a high rating on the stress scale is detected, the clinician can elicit additional information by stating: "There are three major categories of stressors: family stress, work-related stress, and self-inflicted stress." The clinician then briefly pauses to await a response. If a response does not ensue, the clinician can follow up by asking, "Which category represents the majority of your stressors?" A discussion most often follows that explains and interrelates each of the categories of afferent generators (Fig. 6–5) explained in Chapter 2. Time spent in this discussion is very valuable and represents the basis from which the clinician can set realistic short- and long-term treatment goals.

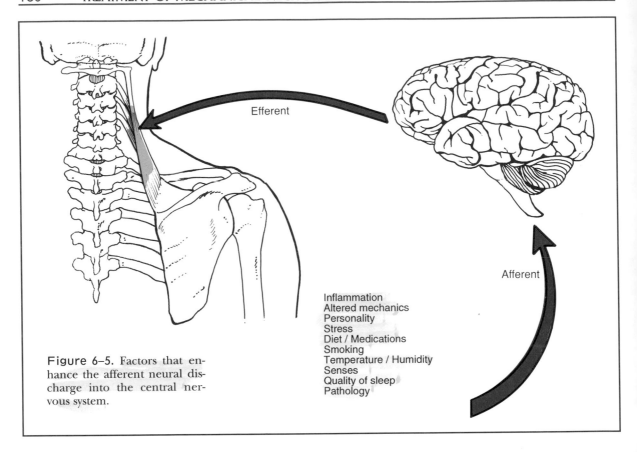

Figure 6–5. Factors that enhance the afferent neural discharge into the central nervous system.

Efferent

Afferent

Inflammation
Altered mechanics
Personality
Stress
Diet / Medications
Smoking
Temperature / Humidity
Senses
Quality of sleep
Pathology

Restoring Anatomical Relations Between Injured and Noninjured Tissues

The next strategy of treatment is to make sure that the injury does not significantly alter function. Depending on a person's pain threshold, an injury can alter movement patterns. This can create overuse syndromes at other sites. A balance must be struck between activity and rest.

Balance between activity and rest is important because it ensures that the injured region does not alter the function of adjacent anatomical regions. This represents a dilemma for the clinician, in that he or she then must make a decision regarding how much activity is enough and how much is excessive with regard to activity and rest. The concept should be that early nondestructive movement is imperative for prompt and com-

plete recovery. The sooner the injured area is moved into a painful range of motion without further injury, the sooner the person recovers. For example, a patient with neck pain that is exacerbated by rotation to the right most often refrains from moving into the painful range. However, during the evaluation, the clinician must make the judgment as to what extent the tissues of the neck can be moved into the painful range without further injury. The successful clinician can obtain patient comfort and confidence so that movement can be carried out into the painful range without exacerbation of the syndrome. This concept assists the patient in minimizing the chances for excessive protective guarding of the area. Early movement enhances normal fluid dynamics and begins to restore normal function. For example, an injury to the apophyseal joint in the neck can lead to a sequence of activities that can alter shoulder function. The central nervous system functions to synchronize muscle contraction about the neck. This results in movement pattern changes of the scapula and humerus.

Maintaining Normal Function of Noninjured Tissue

One of the main factors that inhibits a successful treatment outcome is when the patient permits his or her condition to interfere significantly with normal activity. If the physical dysfunction is accompanied by depression, the syndrome can result in the development of illness behavior.[9, 10] The patient's past experiences with pain and individual interpretation of the meaning of pain are two factors that are intrinsic to illness behavior. The clinician should recognize these interrelationships and set goals accordingly. Two of the clinician's main roles are to assist the patient in performing activities that maintain movement in surrounding tissues and to establish a positive physical and emotional environment.

Preventing Excessive Strain on the Injured Area

The next strategy of treatment for upper-quarter disorders is to assist the patient in completing activities of daily living without further injury. Patients must recognize that to be treated for 1 hour per day 3 days per week represents approximately 5 per cent of the time that they are awake and active. To ensure successful management of the condition, the treatment process should not and cannot stop at the clinic door. The patient must recognize that overuse and exacerbation of the injury are not responses of one activity or event but rather the accumulation of forces into and through the injured region. Judgments relating activities at home or communications with the employer regarding restrictions at work are essential. Protection against overuse during recovery is important. The clinician should be able to recognize overuse by changes in the parameters of the pain pattern, such as increased morning stiffness and changes in protective guarding.

Success of treatment and the quality of recovery from an upper-quarter disorder depend on the understanding of this balance. The injured area requires rest from function to heal and movement to sustain health.

Optimizing Cost-Effectiveness

As the health care industry continues to change, the clinician must recognize that the third party reimburser for medical care is seeking health care services that are efficient and cost-effective. The successful practitioner of the future is the one who becomes skillful in the delivery of a practical active treatment approach based on education that places the patient in the position of taking responsibility for the outcome. The patient must become an educated health care consumer.

An educated health care consumer actively participates in the diagnostic and treatment process. Such a consumer should ask the following questions.

Do I have an understandable diagnosis? The patient should receive and be satisfied with the explanation regarding the diagnosis. A clinician should not make the judgment that the patient cannot comprehend the diagnosis. Placing a name to a condition without a clear explanation often leads to unanswered questions and anxiety. This situation can become amplified if there is disagreement among clinicians involved in the patient's care. To establish the proper role of the patient in the recovery process, the clinician should spend time to make sure that the patient comprehends the diagnosis.

Has an active treatment plan been established? Prolonged passive treatment that does not involve movement in the form of therapeutic exercise may realize short-term positive results but sends the wrong message to the patient and often does not result in long-term benefits.

The questions arise as to whether we can help those patients who do not want to help themselves and should treatment be continued. The initial judgment should be that the patient has a vested interest in maximizing the potential to improve his or her condition. Treatment should be introduced based on that judgment. After a few treatments, the clinician should be able to accurately assess the patient's willingness to participate in the outcome. If the patient has overriding factors likely to hinder treatment progress, then appropriate referral should be made. Persistent, unending treatment of a neuromuscular or musculoskeletal condition without established goals and proper focus represents the nemesis of the medical treatment system. The educated health care consumer desires an active treatment approach that does not render him or her dependent on any health care professional.

Are treatment goals developed and explained? As previously discussed, short- and long-term treatment goals must be established and explained in such a way that the patient is placed in a responsible position. The clinician should assume that the patient wants to improve and return to function as soon as possible. Treatment should not be initiated without the appropriate explanation as to the expected outcomes and time frames. Patients who are uninterested in information should be suspect as to their intentions and motivations.

Do you feel an integral part of the process? To control the escalation of health care costs regarding outpatient services in the future, third party payers will probably institute programs that reward educated health care consumers who pursue this type of treatment behavior and direct their contracts with health care practitioners who practice by a proactive philosophy, that is, prompt, accurate diagnosis of the condition and active treatment programs designed to treat the patient as little as needed to reach the desired goals.

Table 6–3. Objectives of Treatment

1. Pain modulation or promotion of analgesia
    Thermo
    Electrical
    Medical
2. Generate controlled forces to promote nondestructive
      movements
    Manual
    Mechanical
      Traction
      Mobilization tables
      Treatment wedges/rolls
      Heel lifts
      External supports
      Crutches/canes/walkers
    Active
      Muscle energy
      Strain/counterstrain
      Extension/flexion protocols
      Contract/relax techniques
    Common Denominator
      Stimulates fluid dynamics
      Influences afferent input into central nervous
        system
        Regulates pain
        Inhibits muscle contraction
      Modifies connective tissue
3. Enhancing neuromuscular and musculoskeletal
      performance
    Maximizing muscles as shock absorbers
    Establishing movement patterns that minimize
      mechanical stresses
4. Biomechanical counseling
    Establishing limits
      Loads (intensity, frequency, duration)
      Positions (minimize destructive movement
        patterns)

OBJECTIVES OF TREATMENT

Now that the treatment strategies are clearly established, the treatment objectives need to be discussed (Table 6–3). Various treatment approaches have been developed and implemented. Many names have been given to these approaches with an assortment of explanations geared toward establishing differences. This has served as the basis for considerable discussion, but no clear resolution regarding the differences in the professions or treatment techniques has been forthcoming. The emphasis of the investigation has now been modified to explore the similarities among the theories contained within the treatment philosophies for upper-quarter syndromes. The following discussion of the objec-

tives of treatment attempts to identify the scientific basis among the similarities of treatment philosophies.

Once the objectives of treatment are established and discussed, a patient classification system will be instituted as a model to determine appropriate treatment for patients with upper-quarter disorders.

Objective No. 1: Pain Modulation or Promotion of Analgesia

The patient enters the clinician's office with one primary goal: to gain control of the pain. Therefore, the first objective of treatment should be to assist the patient in minimizing the experience of pain. Patients who respond rapidly to pain management treatment have the greatest success in the treatment process. These patients can enter the movement phase of treatment more rapidly and, as a result, can realize a training effect much quicker. Most patients with upper-quarter injuries reach their long-term goals by means of increases in strength, coordination, and endurance of the neuromusculoskeletal system.

Patients who require a more gradual, less aggressive approach to accomplish the desired goals must be managed cautiously. The clinician must guard against patients who place the responsibility for their treatment outcome on the medical profession and anticipate feel-good therapy rather than searching for the appropriate intervention and information to gain control of their conditions. The clinician should be sensitive to their needs and treat appropriately yet gradually proceed to establish the focus of the long-term results of treatment toward self-management. This is accomplished by education and activities that contribute to improved health.

The clinician who teaches the patient population to reach their short- and long-term health goals will be most successful, especially as the population continues to improve their understanding of health. The outpatient office is the place where the public should come for short-term treatment and education; it should also be the place to come with questions regarding overall health. The clinician is in the best position to be the most effective health care educator because he or she interacts with a captive audience: those with pain. Pain influences behavior changes, and long-term successful management of the painful syndrome most often is a function of improved overall health. Therefore, prompt application of appropriate modalities to regulate pain permits the progression toward those treatment objectives and behavioral changes that are responsible for reaching the long-term goal of a painless, active life-style.

Pain Treatment Techniques

Pain can be modulated by several methods of treatment: thermomodalities, electromodalities, and medications.

Thermomodalities. Providing short-term analgesic effects with the use of heat and ice has been advocated for many years as an initial treatment technique. The use of heat and ice in syndromes of the upper quarter have clinical benefit and probably alter the pain-spasm-pain cycle. This initial alteration of the neurophysiology of pain often is needed to initiate successful management of the syndrome. The patient enters in pain, and these modalities are quite effective in the alteration of intensity of that sensation. Which modality is best is questionable. Heat applied to a new injury can theoretically create an increase in the syndrome. However, heat application can best provide muscle relaxation. Conversely, the initial application of ice to an injury is advocated to control the inflammatory process by decreasing the fluid dynamics and the metabolism of the cells. Yet ice applied to the neck region sometimes can exacerbate the syndrome. Therefore, the same rule should be implemented as for injuries to other parts of the body: use ice initially if tolerated and then progress to the use of heat. Topical application of a thermomodality can positively affect the afferent barrage of the nervous system and alter the fluid dynamic and has been effective for many years in the clinical setting at the beginning of the treatment process. The patient should be informed that thermomodalities are used as a temporary means to control pain and should not be thought of as the foundation for long-term management.

Electromodalities. The use of electricity in the treatment of musculoskeletal disorders has been an integral part of the medical field for many years, with effects purported to be minimization of pain and enhancement of fluid dynamics. As with thermomodalities, electrotherapies should be used conservatively in the initial phases of pain management. Although the scientific basis for their action is not fully understood, it is clear that their use helps to modulate pain. For acute problems in the upper quarter, microcurrent, especially using probes, is effective for rapid pain management. This is only one of many techniques that can be used for electrotherapy. Patients should recognize that the effects are temporary with this type of treatment and that the only long-term result is developing the understanding and the knowledge to care for the condition on their own.

A logical explanation for the positive effects of

electromodalities is the disruption of the pain-spasm-pain cycle by means of stimulation of the afferent neural pathways that inhibit the protective guarding mechanisms that optimize tissue fluid dynamics. The clinician should recognize that because the patient's chief complaint is pain, he or she should use whatever combination of modalities that best ameliorates the perception of pain. The decision as to what modality is to be used is based somewhat on the phase of healing but also on clinician preference. Short-term desensitization of a painful region is often not a difficult process. However, its effect on the long-term outcome is questionable. The accepted use of these modalities is to desensitize the painful area for the purpose of enhancing the healing potential and the early introduction of therapeu-

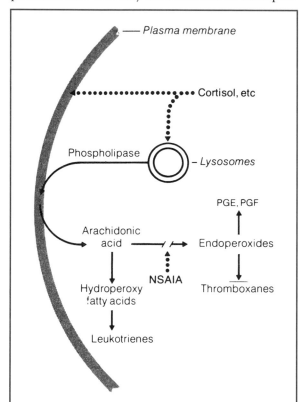

Figure 6–6. Chemical changes associated with cell wall (phospholipid) breakdown. Note that the NSAIDs are designed to block the production of endoperoxides, thereby decreasing the vasodilation action of prostaglandins. (From Weissmann G: Current Concepts. Upshaw Co, 1980, p 26.)

tic exercise. They should not be used primarily as the basis of treatment.

Medications. The medications used to manage upper-quarter syndromes are nonsteroidal anti-inflammatory drugs (NSAIDs), muscle relaxants, analgesics, and, occasionally, psychotherapeutic medications. Figures 6–7 through 6–9 show the classification of the medications used for these problems. The medications are presented in this way so that the clinician can become familiar with the names, categories, and uses of medications prescribed for patients with upper-quarter disorders. The list will be revised and amended as our knowledge of their use and new products are developed.

NSAIDs. NSAIDs are used to block the production of a strong vasodilator, prostaglandin. Figure 6–6 shows the breakdown of the cell wall (phospholipid) as a result of injury, which leads to the formation of arachidonic acid. Further biochemical reactions result in the formation of leukotrienes (chemotaxic agents), prostaglandins (many purposes, one of which is vasodilation), and thromboxanes (induce platelet aggregation). These biochemical reactions are normal, and nonsteroidal medications are designed to block the prostaglandin formation to minimize the osmotic pressure inherent in the inflammatory process.

The introduction of a NSAID is effective in some patients. The physician usually prescribes a particular medication based on previous experience, recognition of potential adverse effects, and personal preference. In general, if a NSAID from one classification is not effective, then another from a different class may be beneficial. Figure 6–7 shows a classification of NSAIDs.

The adverse effects of short- and long-term NSAID use need to be recognized. They include gastritis, possible kidney damage, liver enzyme changes, and central nervous system disturbances, such as vertigo and tinnitus. Although prostaglandin is responsible for the chemical balance of an injury, it also serves to inhibit hydrochloric acid production in the stomach. The prolonged use of NSAIDs can cause an increase in the production of hydrochloric acid; an imbalance of hydrochloric acid can dissolve the mucosal lining of the stomach and diminish its pro-

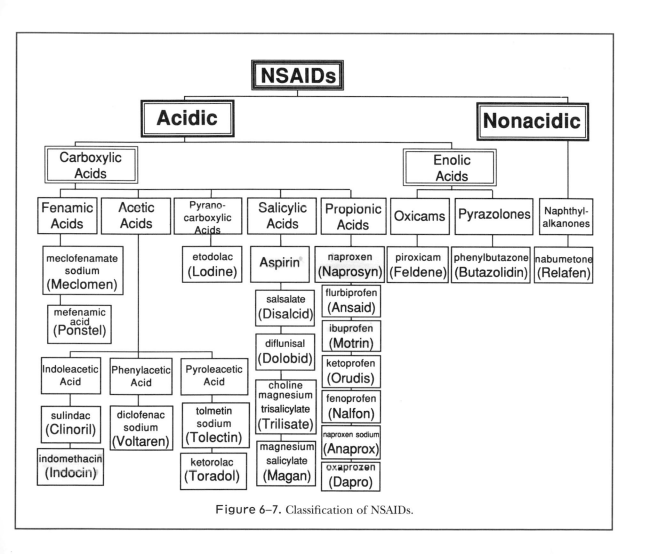

Figure 6–7. Classification of NSAIDs.

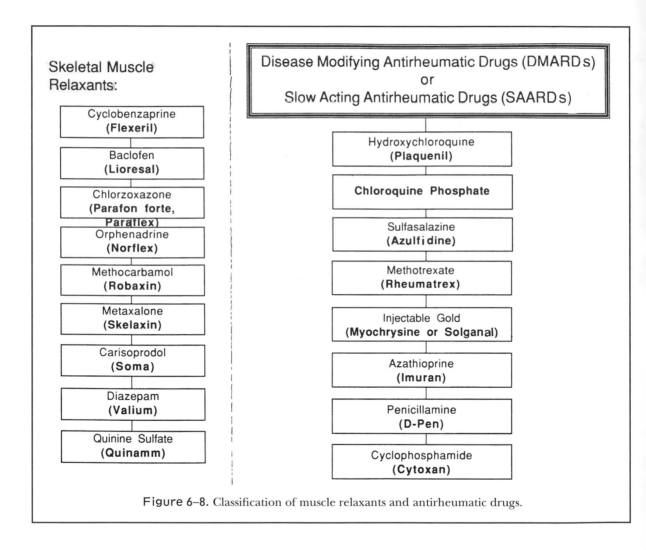

Figure 6–8. Classification of muscle relaxants and antirheumatic drugs.

tective qualities. Acid indigestion is a common complaint of a patient using NSAIDs. If this occurs, the prescribing physician should be notified.

Longstanding usage of NSAIDs can also render the kidneys vulnerable to damage. Prostaglandin is used by the kidneys for vasodilation. Prolonged inhibition of vasodilation of the kidneys can also lead to tissue damage. The patient should be aware of the possible adverse effects of any prescribed drug, and the clinician must be cognizant as to the intended use, desired outcomes, and potential adverse effects.

Some NSAIDs require monitoring of liver enzymes because their use may alter liver biochemistry and must, therefore, be discontinued.

Muscle Relaxants. The purpose of using muscle relaxants in the treatment of upper-quarter or other musculoskeletal or neuromuscular conditions commonly seen in the outpatient clinic is to decrease muscle spasm. Muscle spasm, especially in a patient who has pain, usually represents protective guarding. Like inflammation, protective guarding should not be thought of as unnecessary, but rather as a necessity to protect the injured region from the introduction of injurious forces and stresses. If pain occurs as a result of prolonged muscle contraction, then the patient should heed that warning as signal to stop the activity and temporarily rest from function. Routine use of muscle relaxants during the day should be carefully assessed. Blocking the ability to sustain muscle contraction during the activities of daily living decreases protective guarding and diminishes the needed warning signal for overuse.

Muscle relaxants have been shown experimentally to depress polysynaptic reflexes, produce sedation, and depress neuronal activity essential for quality function.[1] Therefore, these medications should be reserved for use only in the evening to enhance sleep. Figure 6–8 classifies muscle relaxants. Figure 6–9 lists commonly used medications for upper-quarter disorders that are analgesics, a combination of nonsteroidal medication and muscle relaxant, and psychotherapeutic medications.

Analgesics. Analgesics can be useful in the short term during the initial phases of the treatment process. Their use is determined by the severity of the injury and the perception of the physician as to the extent of disability caused by the pain.

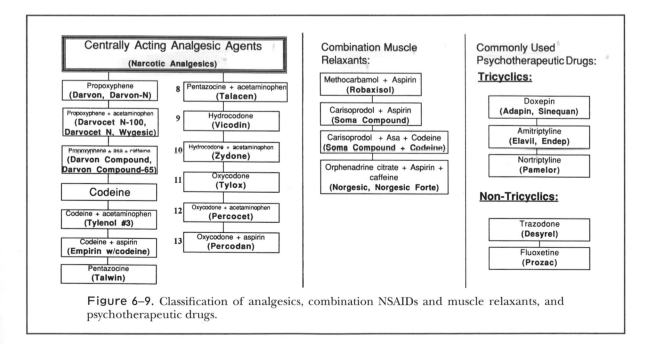

Figure 6–9. Classification of analgesics, combination NSAIDs and muscle relaxants, and psychotherapeutic drugs.

The extent of their use is a good indicator of the severity of pain and the patient's coping ability. One of the initial goals of treatment is to use the minimal effective dose of analgesics and to monitor and eventually taper their use.

Objective No. 2: Generate Controlled Forces to Promote Nondestructive Movements

An important tenet of treating musculoskeletal disorders is that early nondestructive movement is essential for healing. Early movement has many benefits; the primary one is to restore function.

The second objective of the treatment process represents another way to alter the painful syndrome by way of gradual, progressive movement. Over the years, various forms of manual therapy have taken on different names with various descriptions of their purported effects. Generating controlled forces through the region can be divided into three categories: manual techniques, mechanical devices, and active and active assistive movement.

Manual Techniques

Included in this category of manual treatment for painful conditions are massage (effleurage, petrissage, tapotement, cross friction, traeger, rolfing), soft tissue mobilization, myofascial techniques, manipulation, traction, stretching, accupressure, and acupuncture. Although the application of the manual techniques may differ, the intended outcomes are similar. Whatever the technique, the patient should be informed as to why it is being used as a treatment modality. The use of manual techniques in the initial stages of the treatment process is important because not only does it assist in altering the afferent neural input, but it is an effective method of maintaining fluid movement (Fig. 6–10).

The following is an example of manual treatment protocols for a patient with a typical upper-quarter syndrome: neck pain worse than arm pain, pain that often is referred into the scapular region and into the arm as the condition worsens, and difficulty with mobility of the neck and in sustaining prolonged postures of sitting and standing. The purposes of this treatment are to increase the afferent input into the central nervous system, assure an increase in fluid dynamics

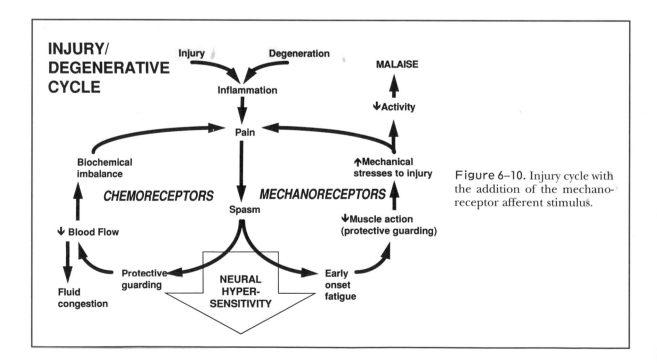

Figure 6–10. Injury cycle with the addition of the mechanoreceptor afferent stimulus.

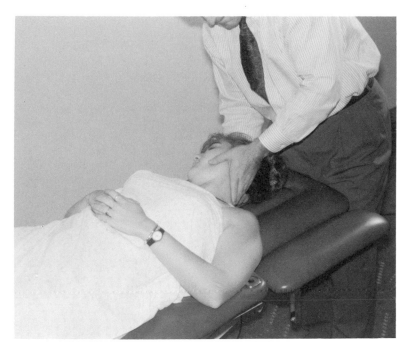

Figure 6–11. Passive rotation to the right. Note the placement of the hands. The head is cradled in the fingers with a firm, even pressure of all the digits. The cradling hand should be relaxed and make as much contact as possible. The other hand is placed on the frontal region and is used to guide motion and direct overpressure.

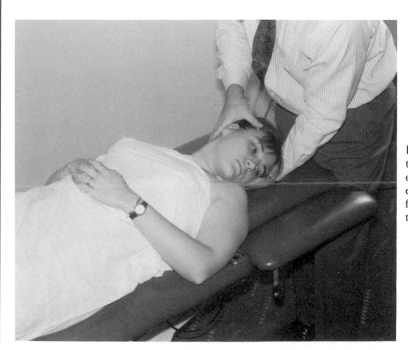

Figure 6–12. Passive rotation to the left. Three or four repetitions can be performed to either side until comfort, confidence, and relaxation are established.

and at the same time gradually move the patient in a controlled manner into the painful range, and outline the barriers of range of motion.

Figures 6–11 through 6–25 depict a manual treatment regimen (sequence) that can be carried out for patients with typical upper-quarter syndromes. The sequence can be rearranged based on clinician preference or assessment findings.

Positioning. To begin the treatment process, the patient should be positioned supine as comfortably as possible. A combination of pillows under the knees or legs or a bolster under the legs that places the hips and knees at about 60 degrees flexion most often suffices. The clinician should be able to adjust the lighting to improve patient comfort. It is difficult to successfully manage most upper-quarter problems under harsh fluorescent lighting. A rheostat can be installed to dim the light or a softer, bluer light can replace the fluorescent bulbs.

Passive Range of Motion. The treatment process can begin by properly and comfortably supporting the head and then performing passive range of motion of the cervical spine first to the right and then to the left (Figs. 6–11 and 6–12). The clinician should assure the patient that no quick and unexpected motions will be used. The clinician continues to move gently, rocking the head into rotation right and left. The clinician uses the findings of the antigravity examination to predict the positions and ranges that are most uncomfortable for the patient.

The patient is then asked to assist in rotation, and the patient then gently resists the motion. The clinician evaluates the barriers felt through the hands and gradually takes the patient toward the available end ranges and evaluates the resistance felt. The use of the neuromuscular techniques described in Chapter 3 are effective in increasing motion.

Soft Tissue Mobilization: Upper Quarter—Supine Position. Treatment continues by placing the head and neck in a neutral position. The treatment can begin by gently stroking the skin bilaterally from the superior medial borders of the scapula to the occiput. This technique is a gentle massage that progresses into manual cer-

vical traction (Fig. 6–13). After several stroking techniques, the clinician grasps the occiput at the end of the stroke and directs traction to the cervical spine. This traction, if tolerated, can be held momentarily, and soft tissue mobilization continues. As the patient relaxes, increased passive motion of the cervical spine often is realized.

From the neutral cervical position, a passive extension force can be imparted to the tissues of the cervical spine (Fig. 6–14). The hands are placed on either side of the cervical spine, and together a force is generated parallel to the apophyseal joint plane. As the force is applied to the cervical spine, the occiput is gently extended.

Once this is completed, the head is supported with the right hand and the left hand is used to provide a stroking technique into rotation to the right. The left hand begins near the superior medial aspect of the scapula, and the stroke proceeds superior as the left and right hands gently rotate the head to the right (Fig. 6–15). This rhythmic activity in a painless range of motion should be relaxing. The clinician should visualize the oblique plane of the apophyseal joints and use the hands to guide the cervical spine through a gentle range of motion. The right hand creates, by way of its position on the occiput, a slow, controlled, repetitive motion.

By adding a traction force with both or either hand, the clinician can apply additional force to the cervical spine. This traction can be directed toward a particular region of the neck by virtue of hand placement and direction of the forces.

Once this is done a number of times, the clinician continues the rhythmic motion by carefully transferring the head from the right hand to the left hand. Jerking, uncoordinated movements should be avoided. Slow, rhythmic, coordinated activity will probably produce the best results by gaining the patient's confidence and avoiding excessive stimulus into the region. The stroking continues with the right hand. Again, beginning at the superior medial border of the scapula, the upward stroke to the cervical spine is coupled with a rotation of the cervical spine to the right. Range of motion is gradually increased until the barrier is found. At any time during this rhythmic activity, the patient is asked to assist in rotation left and right. Active, controlled muscle contraction is one of the most efficient ways to stimulate relaxation and enhance fluid dynamics.

Text continued on page 195

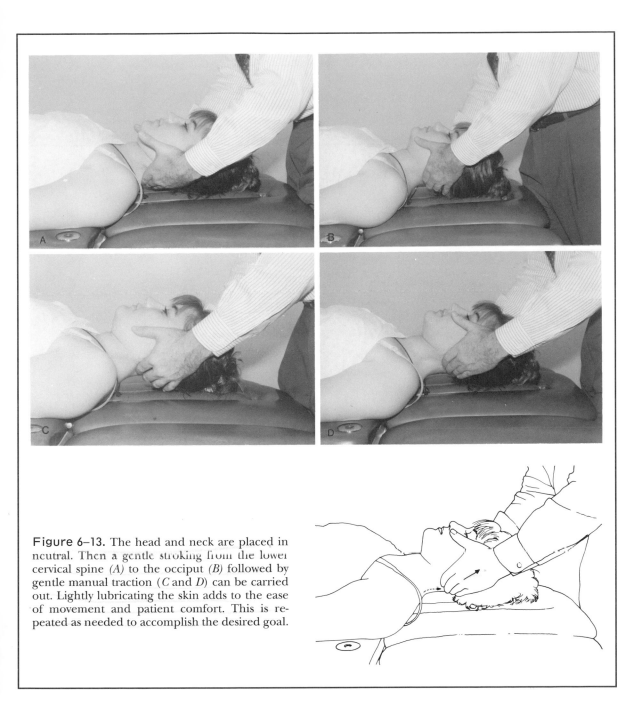

Figure 6–13. The head and neck are placed in neutral. Then a gentle stroking from the lower cervical spine (*A*) to the occiput (*B*) followed by gentle manual traction (*C* and *D*) can be carried out. Lightly lubricating the skin adds to the ease of movement and patient comfort. This is repeated as needed to accomplish the desired goal.

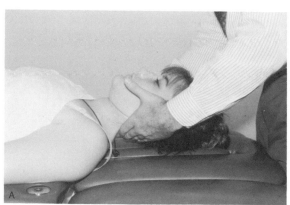

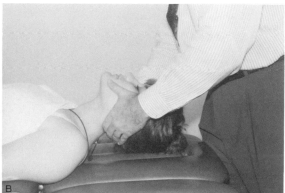

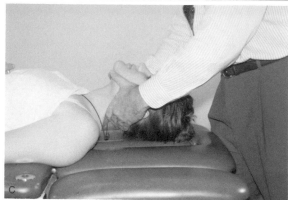

Figure 6–14. Starting with the neck in neutral position and at the lower cervical spine *(A)*, a gentle passive extension can be carried out *(B)*. The extension force imparted to the spine should be directed along the 45-degree apophyseal joint plane. Once the hands reach the occiput, a gentle extension moment can be directed to the occiput and cervical spine. The clinician can pause at any position and create passive extension by gently permitting the occiput to tilt backward while the index fingers of the examiner's hands are lifting anteriorly and superiorly (extension) *(C)*.

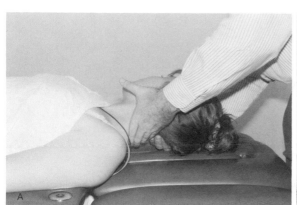
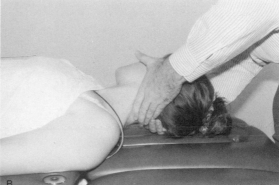
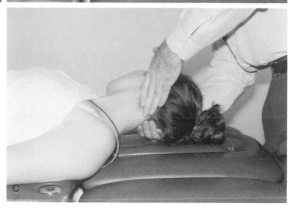

Figure 6–15. The treatment continues by repeating passive rotation to the right and is augmented by stroking of the skin. This technique should begin near the superior medial border of the scapula *(A)* and progress to the mastoid process region *(B* and *C)* as the passive rotation is carried out. The clinician easily searches for the barrier—that point at which the nociceptor depolarizes. It may take a number of repetitions to reach that range of motion. The barrier often changes as the other repetitions follow. The clinician should not be in haste to identify the painful barrier and should cautiously enter the painful range.

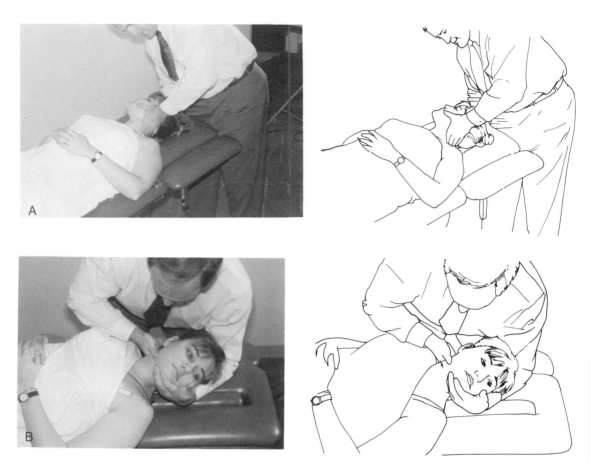

Figure 6–16. Like the assessment process, combination movements can be performed to enhance mobility of the cervical spine. In this example *(A)*, the examiner is using the right hand to position the occiput into right rotation and cervical side bending to the left while the left hand imparts a force to the mid cervical spine as if to move the inferior articulating process of the vertebra above up in a 45-degree direction on the superior articulating process of the vertebrae below. This combination movement slowly takes that segment to end range. The mobilization force should be generated by way of the concepts of graded mobilization outlined by Geoffrey Maitland.[6] Another position can be used to accomplish a similar means *(B)*. In this position, the clinician cradles the patient's head in the left hand and forearm while the clinician's right metacarpophalangeal joint and index finger directs the force along the joint plane.

After completion of this stroking technique first to the right and then the left, the clinician can use a combination of movements and forces to augment mobilization of the cervical spine (Fig. 6–16). These techniques are designed specifically to direct end-range forces to a cervical segment. They are carried out in a gradual and progressive manner, depending on the injury (swelling) status of the tissue.[6] High-velocity, short thrusting is not indicated in the cervical spine. Full range of motion to end range can be effectively carried out if the amplitude and direction of the forces are properly conducted.

Figure 6–16A shows a technique that mobilizes the left mid cervical spine by rotation to the right and side bending to the left, while the right hand generates a force anterior and superior along the 45-degree apophyseal joint plane. This combination of positions and movements subject that seg-

ment to end range. Figure 6–16B shows another technique that specifically generates a superior and anterior force to the right mid cervical region. Either technique can be used to stimulate fluid movement and afferent input into the central nervous system.

If sustained manual traction is preferred, the clinician can use a mobilization strap to augment the technique (Fig. 6–17). The strap is placed around the clinician's mid sacral region and looped around each hand. The clinician's hands firmly and completely grasp the patient's occiput and cranium. Grasping the cranium in this manner can compress the patient's ears, so earrings should be removed. For patients who may be uncomfortable about having their ears covered, an explanation as to what is about to follow may be indicated. Patient comfort is imperative.

Once the head is comfortably positioned, a

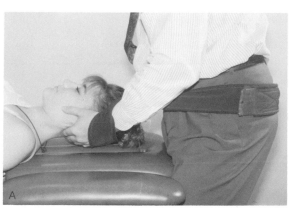
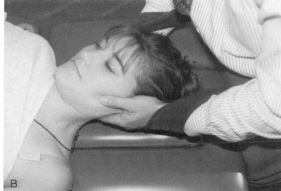
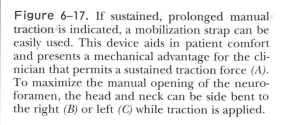
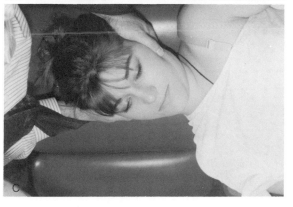

Figure 6–17. If sustained, prolonged manual traction is indicated, a mobilization strap can be easily used. This device aids in patient comfort and presents a mechanical advantage for the clinician that permits a sustained traction force (A). To maximize the manual opening of the neuroforamen, the head and neck can be side bent to the right (B) or left (C) while traction is applied.

gentle, direct midrange pull is performed. The clinician may want to begin with intermittent traction of short duration before a sustained traction. Figure 6–17A shows a direct midrange traction. With the strap, the clinician merely moves the pelvis in a posterior direction to augment the pull. The strap greatly improves the mechanics of the pull, thereby minimizing fatigue and improving patient comfort. Figure 6–17B and C (side bending to the right and to the left, respectively) illustrate sustained traction in a side-bent position. This position directs the force to the convex side, which increases the opening or widening aspect of the neuroforamen. The assessment findings determine the desired position of the treatment.

Soft Tissue Mobilization: Upper Quarter— Right Side-Lying Position. The patient is then comfortably positioned right side-lying (Fig. 6–18) so that mobilization of the upper quarter can continue. Figure 6–19 shows a treatment sequence performed to carry out the goals and objectives previously described. These techniques are effective in creating patient comfort and decreasing pain.

The passive, active assistive, or active resistive mobilization of the upper quarter can continue by changing the direction of movements, as shown in Figure 6–20. This alteration in movement patterns will further stimulate the afferent nervous system and alter the fluid dynamics of the upper quarter.

The mobilization continues by altering the movement pattern to include a circular motion. The technique, as outlined in Figure 6–21, shows a clockwise sequence. It is suggested that the movement initially be carried out passively, progressing to active assistive and then to active resistive exercise. The sooner the patient can be involved in the movement, the greater the chances for reaching the desired goal. The clinician must judge the extent of the patient's involvement by the injury status. Morning stiffness, stiffness experienced after prolonged postures, and tissue tenderness are the best determinants of tissue

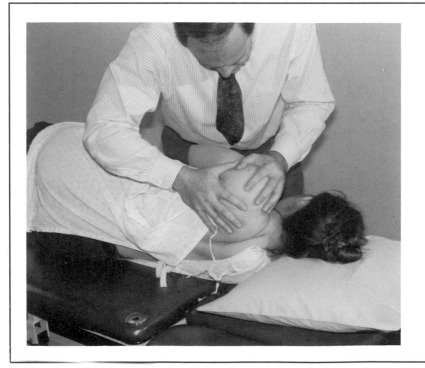

Figure 6–18. Starting position for right side-lying mobilization. A pillow is placed between the patient's legs and under the head. The spine should be placed in a neutral position. The table height is raised so that the clinician is positioned directly over the humerus with the left hand controlling the acromium and humeral head and the right hand controlling the scapula.

damage. Relaxation is best accomplished as active movement is introduced.

As the movement becomes free and un-impeded, the opposite direction (counterclock-wise) should be performed. Repetitions and sets depend on the time and variation of the treatment sequence necessary to accomplish the goal.

The side-lying treatment of upper-quarter conditions includes specific soft tissue massage (Fig. 6–22). The side-lying position provides an easy access to the tissues that are most often involved in the upper-quarter syndrome. Movement of the upper quarter as previously described followed by soft tissue mobilization of the tissues complement each other and augment the treatment program.

The technique includes passive motion and associated stroking of the tissues. This mobilization technique is effective in creating fluid changes in the region and permits specific work at the origin of the levator scapulae. Tenderness in this area in patients with upper quarter dysfunction often is caused by overuse of this strong cervical spine stabilizer. The previous treatment regimen provides excellent results with respect to relaxation and nondestructive stimulation to the afferent nervous system. This type of treatment is designed to desensitize the nervous system by altering the efferent (motor) gain by stimulation to the afferent system. This stimulation modulates pain, stimulates fluid dynamics, and regulates the state of muscle contraction.

Soft Tissue Mobilization: Upper Quarter— Left Side-Lying Position. The patient is then asked to lie on the opposite side so that the same type of activity can be repeated to the left scapulothoracic region.

Manual Traction and Tissue Mobilization: Upper Quarter—Seated Position. Another manual technique to generate controlled forces to the upper quarter can be performed in a seated position. Although manual traction can be administered in this position (Fig. 6–23), the seated position is best used if the clinician is attempting to increase range of motion of the cervical spine by passive mobilization. Figures 6–24 and 6–25 show techniques for generating rotational and extension forces to the cervical spine. Other tech-niques are also effective at altering fluid dynamics and modulating pain and muscle contraction.[2, 3]

The previous treatment sequence is an example of a global technique that can affect the soft tissues of the upper quarter. During the sequence, the clinician can educate the patient as to expected outcomes, discuss home treatment programs, and revamp short-term goals.

A major portion of the home program is to ensure two or three episodes of short-term rest at home. The patient is encouraged to decrease all stimuli, such as radio and television and harsh lights, and then adopt the most comfortable position possible so that he or she can relax for at least 5 minutes. Unloading the neck and upper quarter by stabilizing the head in a comfortable position is an excellent way to assist these tissues in resting against function, and it forces the patient to break up the day, which minimizes the chances for initiating the pain-spasm-pain cycle.

Because many types of tissues can be affected during mobilization, one should avoid taking the neck to end range with excessive force. Repetitive end-range motion usually is not indicated and should only be used by those who have perfected the skill. Manipulation affords a way to rapidly alter the pain-spasm-pain cycle by means of brisk afferent input into the central nervous system. These techniques are temporarily effective in causing relaxation and decreasing pain. However, manipulation techniques should only be used short term to facilitate early active motion by the patient and then discontinued as the treatment program progresses by shifting the onus of control from the clinician to the patient. Any treatment that places the clinician in total control so that the patient is dependent on that treatment is not indicated.

Mechanical Means to Introduce Controlled Forces

Different mechanical devices in the form of traction machines, mobilization tables, cervical pillows, and cervical collars can be used to control the forces through the cervical spine and to assist in minimizing forces that can place excessive strain on the injured area. Figure 6–26 shows typical mechanical cervical traction. The goal is to assist the patient in decreasing the compressive

Text continued on page 208

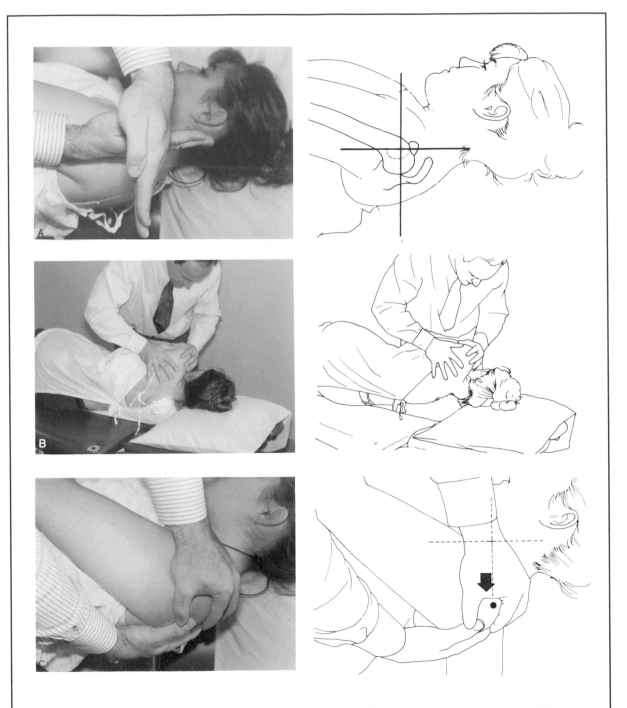

Figure 6–19. From this position, the clinician can visualize an axis (cross) with arms at 90 degrees (A) as they bisect the humeral head. This represents the directions of passive and/or active assistive movements that are about to take place. (B) Hand placements with the left hand at the humeral head and the right hand at the scapula. The sequence commences by retracting the scapula (C).

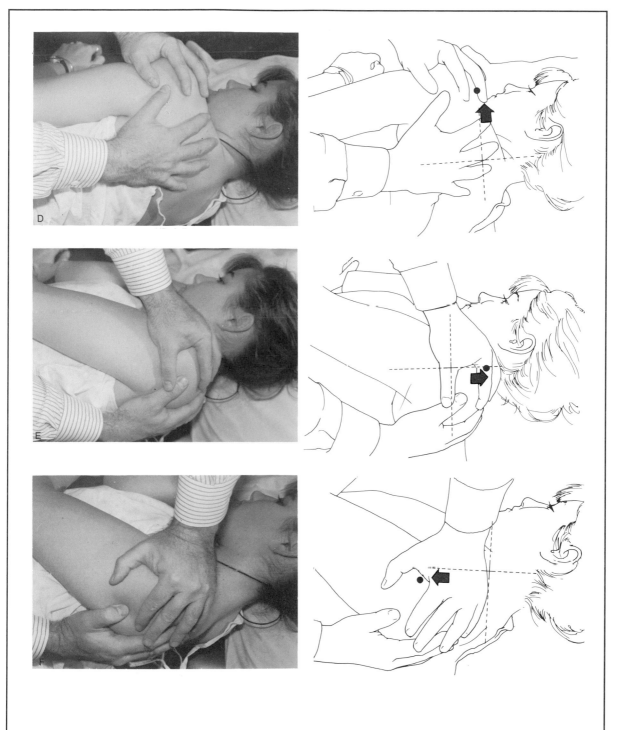

Figure 6–19 *Continued (D)* Retractors of the scapula. This can be followed by passively or actively assisted movement of the scapula along the vertical axis (i.e., elevation [*E*] and then depression [*F*]).

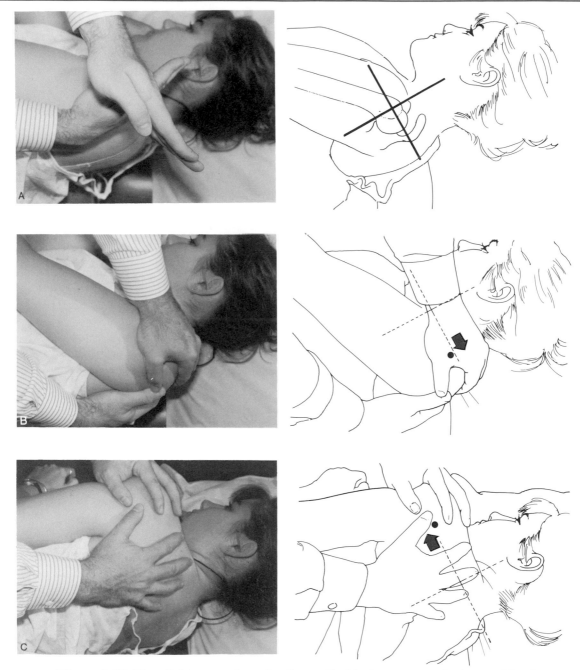

Figure 6–20. The clinician can then visualize an X with the center at the humeral head (A). The passive and/or active assistive manual treatment can continue by moving the scapulo-humeral region in varying patterns: elevated and retracted (B), depressed and protracted (C), elevated and protracted (D), and depressed and retracted (wide view to show position [E] and closed up [F]).

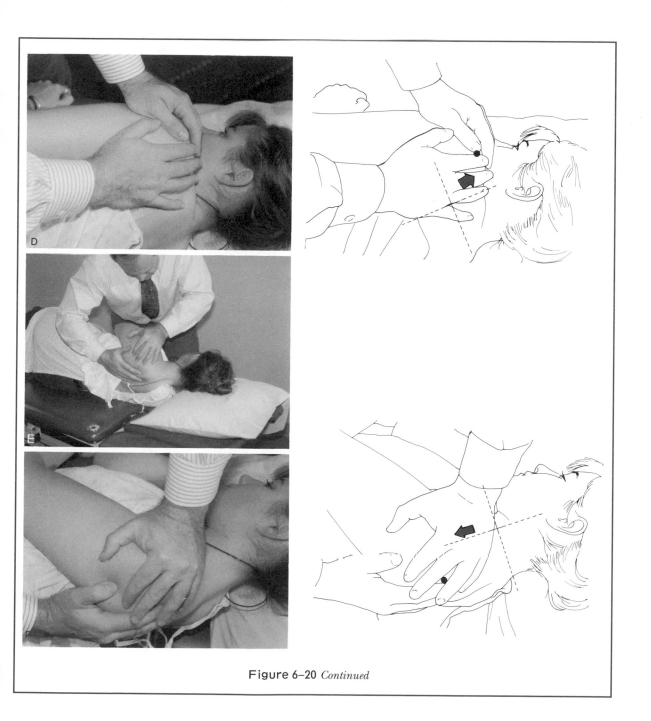

Figure 6-20 *Continued*

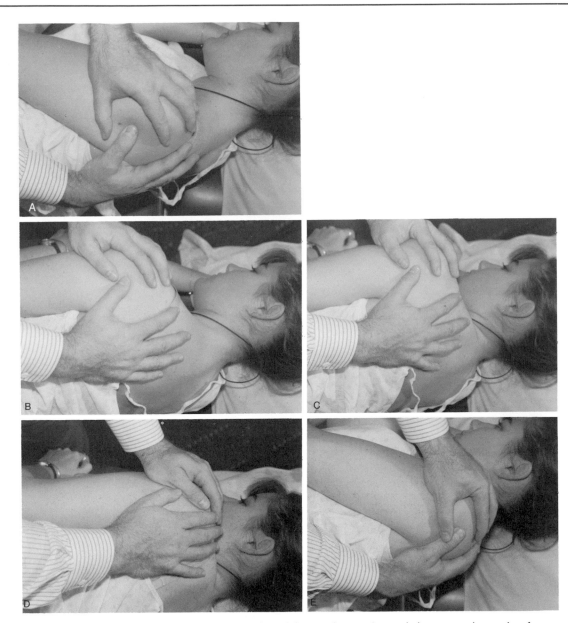

Figure 6–21. Treatment can be continued by passive, active assistive, or active resisted motion in a circular manner. *(A)* Starting position. Sequence moves clockwise. The number of repetitions and sets depends on the individual.

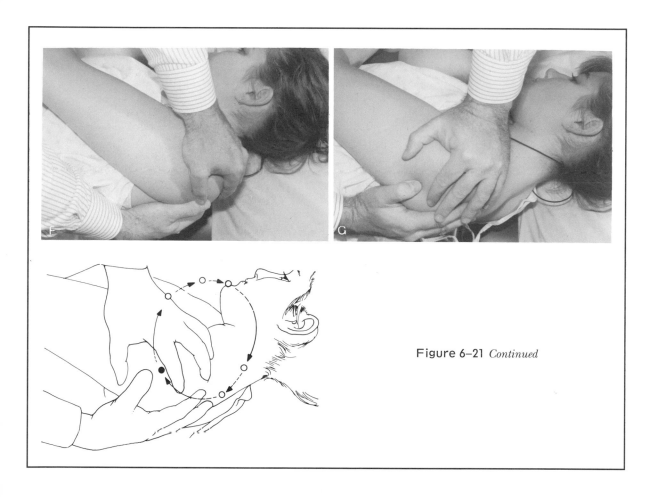

Figure 6–21 *Continued*

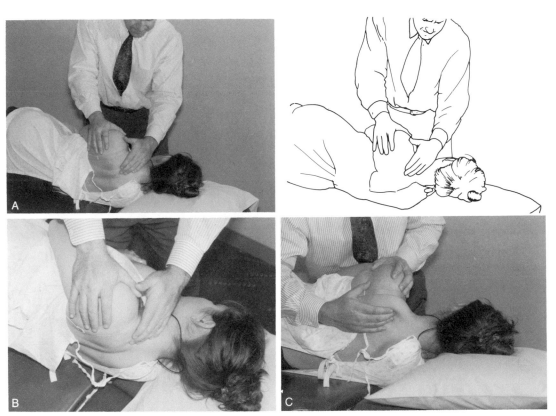

Figure 6–22. Conclusion of right side-lying manual treatment. (*A* and *B*) Gentle stroking superior and anterior by the left hand as the right hand gently retracts the scapula. This rhythmic motion can affect any of the posterior tissues of the upper quarter. (*C*) Specific mobilization of the superior medial border of the scapula (a common site of tenderness) by the left hand as the right hand stabilizes the humerus and acromium.

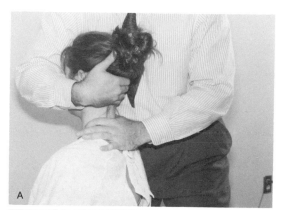

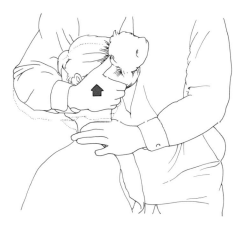

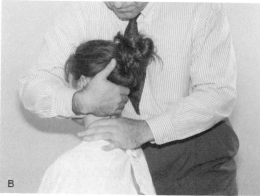

Figure 6–23. Seated position for manual cervical traction. *(A)* The patient's head is stabilized against the clinician's chest. The clinician grasps the occiput with the right index finger and extends the hand down to the segment to which the traction is to be directed (little finger). The left hand grasps the base of the cervical spine. *(B)* The clinician generates a traction force by pulling up with the chest and right hand while pushing down with the left hand.

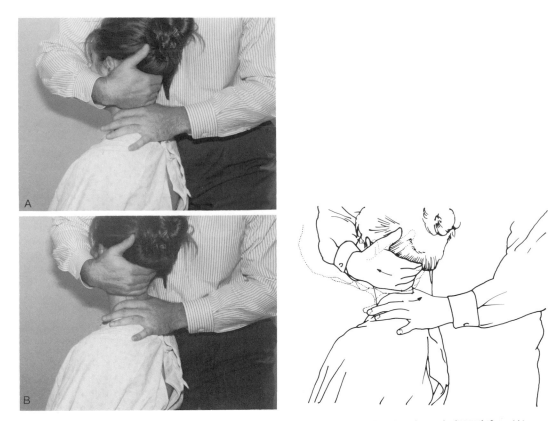

Figure 6–24. Seated position for mobilization of the cervical spine in rotation right. *(A)* The little finger of the right hand is placed along the segment to which the force is to be generated. The remainder of the right hand is placed on the neck, and the palm grasps the occiput and mastoid process. The index finger and thumb of the left hand grasp below the targeted segment. *(B)* The left hand directs a left rotation force from below and fixates or stops while the right hand applies a right rotation force anterior and superior in a 45-degree direction along the apophyseal joint plane. The force is in equal and opposite directions. The clinician should visualize the left inferior articulating process moving up on the left superior articulating process at the level designated by the hand placements.

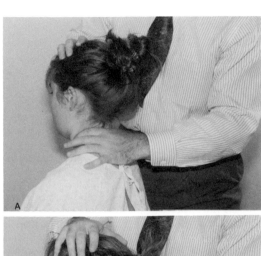
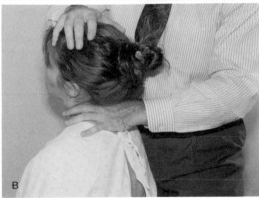
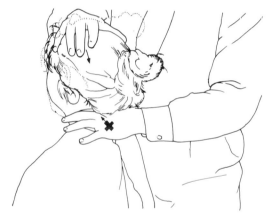

Figure 6–25. Seated position for mobilization of the cervical spine in extension. *(A)* The clinician's right hand is placed on the right frontal aspect of the patient's head. The left hand, particularly the index finger, is placed at the targeted segment. *(B)* The mobilization begins by using the index finger of the left hand as a fixed point by creating an anterior and superior force (along the 45-degree apophyseal joint plane) to the articular pillar of the vertebrae. This force creates a small rotation to the right. With the left hand fixed, the right hand applies a backward bending and side bending to the left force. The combination of forces converge just above the fixed point to cause the inferior articulating process of the vertebra above to move down and back on the vertebra below.

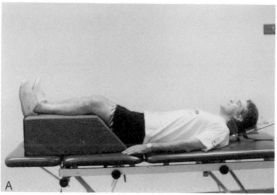

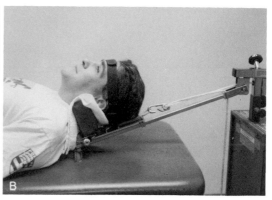

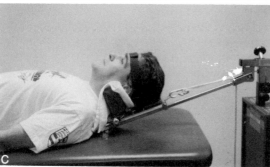

Figure 6–26. Mechanical cervical traction. *(A)* Proper positioning with the hips and knees flexed and stabilized. *(B)* Utilization of a mechanical traction device where the occiput is stabilized on either side by an adjustable pad, and the head is secured by a strap. *(C)* Traction is either applied intermittently or sustained, and the duration is dependent on clinician preference. The traction force must be at least the weight of the head.

forces imparted to the cervical spine, thereby decreasing the afferent input into the central nervous system and altering the pain-spasm-pain cycle.

Figure 6–27 shows the use and modification of the foam cervical collar as a common device used to immobilize the head and neck. Temporarily used, this device can be effective in the initial phases of the treatment process for disorders of the upper quarter. Cervical collars are available in three sizes. Some modification may be necessary to maximize the proper fit. Sizing the cervical collar depends on the neck size and the position and forces that exacerbate the familiar symptoms. For example, if the patient has a small neck and backward bending increases the symptoms, then the collar can either be adapted to fit the chin by cutting out the front to properly po-

sition the head or be turned around so that the narrow end fastens in the front.

Active Techniques. To generate controlled forces into the area, active techniques often are used to enhance the healing process. Like manual techniques, there are many names for these activities, such as muscle energy, strain-counterstrain, extension and flexion protocols, and contract-relax techniques. Using contraction of the muscle to increase the afferent input into the nervous system and enhance fluid dynamics is important in the overall scope of treatment. Again, the goal of this objective is to generate controlled forces, and the clinician must decide the intensity, frequency, and duration of these forces so as not to further the injury process. These active techniques are designed to promote

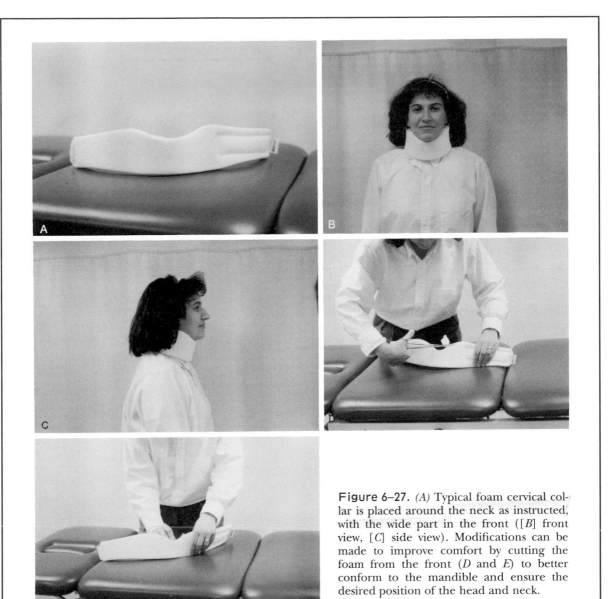

Figure 6–27. (*A*) Typical foam cervical collar is placed around the neck as instructed, with the wide part in the front ([*B*] front view, [*C*] side view). Modifications can be made to improve comfort by cutting the foam from the front (*D* and *E*) to better conform to the mandible and ensure the desired position of the head and neck.

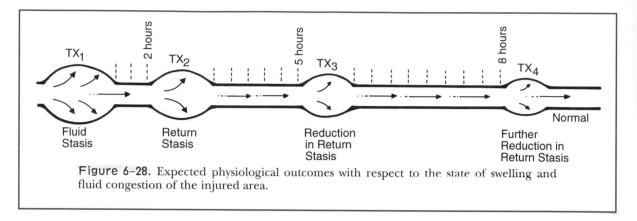

Figure 6–28. Expected physiological outcomes with respect to the state of swelling and fluid congestion of the injured area.

muscle contraction in a nondestructive range of motion, which is important in neutralizing normal function of the injured area.

The common denominator among all these techniques is that they stimulate fluid dynamics, which includes both blood flow and lymph drainage, and the techniques stimulate afferent input in the central nervous system. This afferent input helps to regulate pain and modulate muscle contraction, which are essential for enhancement of normal biomechanics and normal function. Manual techniques are important in the initial onset of treatment of musculoskeletal disorders, especially in the upper quarter, and can be effective in decreasing the many parameters of the syndrome.

Figure 6–28 diagrams the expected result of the techniques outlined within this objective of treatment. Treatment to alter fluid dynamics is designed to enhance the healing time and progress toward functional repair. As the treatment is given, venous flow and lymph drainage are stimulated and temporary relief of pain and stiffness (swollen state) is expected. The rate at which the swollen state reappears is indicative of the extent of the injury. The more significant the injury, the quicker the return of fluid. This information is important for the clinician who is attempting to determine the progression of treatment. The quicker the return to the pretreatment state of feeling (stiffness and pain), the slower the progression. Figure 6–28 shows the expected outcome, that is, a slower return to a lesser extent of the pretreatment state of swelling. This type of treatment enhances the physiology of healing connective tissues. Progressing toward

activities that restore function and education for self-management is the goal.

Objective No. 3: Enhancing Neuromuscular and Musculoskeletal Performance

The synchronization of muscle contraction is important in controlling the way in which the specialized connective tissues attenuate forces. Muscles greatly assist in attenuating these forces. In the upper quarter, it is important that muscle contraction be synchronized in a manner that minimally causes compression and tensile forces to all the tissues in the neck. It is also important that the clinician assist the patient in recognizing the movement patterns that minimize unwanted or destructive stresses into the upper quarter and proceed accordingly. Increasing the strength, power, and endurance of the upper-quarter musculature so that the forces of the head can be counterbalanced throughout the day as well as enhancing those activities performed by the arms and scapula are the ultimate goals. Strengthening is crucial to stimulate tissue growth and minimize reinjury. The most efficient and productive way to reach this goal is to follow the principles discussed below. These principles are designed to maximize the training effect and at the same time improve the coordination and motor learning required to effectively carry out the activities of living for both work and recreation.

Utilize Submaximal Workloads in Leading to Progressive Resistance Exercises (Overload). Using the information gained from the assessment process, the clinician can begin to design a therapeutic exercise program that will maximize the use of the muscles as shock absorbers and to develop movement patterns that do not exacerbate the injury. This process is begun by using submaximal workloads. Initially during the therapeutic exercise training program, the clinician should focus on teaching the principles of establishing safe and complete movement patterns and at the same time begin to stimulate strength, power, and endurance of the musculature. Unlike in the low back, where hypertrophy and high force production are the ultimate goals, the musculature of the neck must react rapidly and be able to endure many prolonged positions of the head and neck.

Stabilization in the form of maintaining proper nondestructive positions while carrying out normal function is the goal for both the low back and the neck. The functions of both differ; therefore, training should be specifically designed to maximize the particular function. In the neck, overload is not the goal for those tissues that specifically attach into the neck, yet for the scapular and chest muscles, hypertrophy and overload apply.

Exercise Until Momentary Fatigue (Repetitions to Substitution). Although asking the patient to perform a particular number of repetitions in the initial phases of the rehabilitation process is indicated, progression toward an understanding of repetitions to substitution is warranted. Repetitions to substitution refers to a focus on the movement pattern being performed rather than on a number of repetitions. Once the patient can learn and adhere to this concept of resistive movement, the chance of reinjury diminishes and the goals of training can be efficiently accomplished.

An example of such a pattern would be the patient who has pain reproduced with backward bending and with backward bending and side bending to the right. In this case, the instruction would be to preposition the head and neck slightly into a forward bend and side bending to the left. The patient can accomplish this by slightly tucking the chin and side bending the neck to the left. The movement associated with therapeutic exercise should be instructed so that the forces that are generated by the resisted

movement do not overload the injured area in backward bending and side bending to the right. Once this position is lost and the movement pattern of the exercise changes because of fatigue (substitution of muscle function), then the exercise bout should cease. To ensure that the patient can train without injury, this concept must be thoroughly understood.

Vary Loads and Angles of Resistance. As mentioned in Chapter 1, the body responds proportionally to the manner in which it is stressed. By varying the loads and angles of resistance, the motor learning and muscle sequencing responsible for controlled motion are best accomplished.

Progress to More Functional Positions. Isolating the muscle and exercising to momentary fatigue are appropriate concepts for the beginning phases of exercise; however, progressing to positions and movements that replicate normal function is preferred. Specificity of training is a strong physiological principle that should be adhered to as the training process advances.

The questions that arise when developing a training program for someone who is attempting to improve his or her health or is recovering from an injury are, How much? How many? How often? and What position?

How Much? Is the best combination 3 sets of 10 repetitions or 6 sets of 14 repetitions? In reality, a fixed number of sets and repetitions may be too much one day and too little the next. This depends on the patient's condition as he or she begins the exercise bout. The decision as to how much should be based on two variables: the perception of the current state of swelling and the training force. The patient needs to be able to appropriately assess the current state of swelling (injury) at the time of exercise. This can be accomplished by recognizing the subtle feelings that define the status of the condition. Morning stiffness, the amount of protective guarding that is present, and the ability to maintain prolonged positions all serve as cues.

The variables change as the recovery process progresses, and an analysis of the current status of the condition is crucial to ensure that the therapeutic exercise is productive and not counterproductive. If the focus remains on a specific number of sets and repetitions, then the chances of rapidly and completely reaching the goals of exercise without injury are minimal. The patient must learn to make the appropriate decisions at the onset of each exercise session. This knowledge permits the patient to train as the variables of the condition deviate. Deviations of swelling pain and stiffness are common during recovery, and the patient needs to be cognizant of those changes and adjust activities accordingly.

Overload should be encouraged but not at the expense of reinjury or exacerbation. This can only be done by proper education and instruction in the training principles and techniques.

How Many? It is advantageous to begin by establishing a number of repetitions with the amount of weight that makes the last repetition somewhat difficult. Low weight with high repetitions (20 to 30) should be initiated. As the patient becomes more aware of the process and the technique improves, the number is de-emphasized and repetitions to momentary fatigue or substitution of muscle function should be encouraged.

How Often? The answer to this question depends on the time required for total recovery. This depends on the state of the healing process and the ease with which the condition varies. If the syndrome is easily altered by activities, then the time to recover is probably more extended. Therefore, training every other day is appropriate. Conversely, if the healing status of the tissues does not easily vary, then training daily is appropriate. As resistance increases without injury, recovery time usually decreases.

Once the rehabilitation program reaches this objective, it should continue for at least 4 weeks. This time frame is based on the understanding of the neurophysiological changes that emerge as a result of the consistent stresses of training.[5, 7] The patient should be encouraged to exercise under supervision for at least 4 weeks so that he or she can obtain the skills and knowledge to make the proper intensity, frequency, and duration decisions as well as realize the training effects. These effects are the changes in the motor-neuronal adaptations that develop in the first 4 weeks of training.

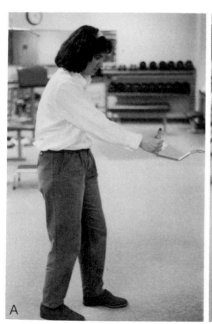 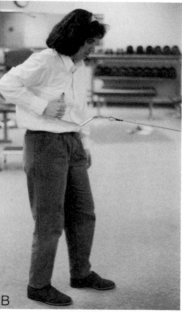

Figure 6–29. *(A)* Starting position for one-arm mid pulls. Before beginning the exercise, the patient should be instructed as to the concepts of training and the position (head, neck, and foot) that needs to be maintained. *(B)* End position for one-arm pull. Note the midrange position of the movement, which minimizes chances for exacerbation.

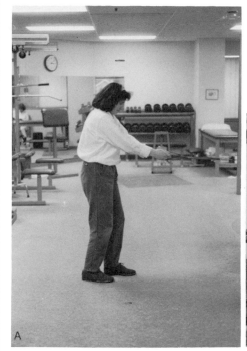
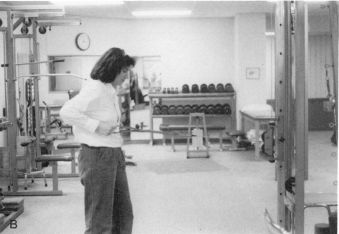

Figure 6–30. *(A)* Starting position for bilateral mid pulls. The patient should maintain the position of the head, neck, and trunk throughout the exercise. *(B)* End position for bilateral mid pulls. Once it has been determined that this exercise stroke is comfortable, the angle of force can be varied by pulling the strap toward the tops of the knees and then the chin.

What Position? Position is determined by the functional assessment findings. They represent those forces and positions that most exacerbate the syndrome or reproduce familiar pain. To determine the best positions for training exercises, the clinician must analyze the biomechanics of each exercise and then make the determination regarding body position and range of motion. Reaching the training effect depends on overload without exacerbation of symptoms.

Figures 6–29 through 6–40 show several exercises that are commonly used in the rehabilitation process of upper-quarter syndromes. The exercises are focused on the posterior scapular muscles and the abdominal wall. These muscle groups are particularly responsible for maintaining the upright posture. The instruction to the patient is to position the head and neck before doing the exercise. The prepositioning selected is based on the assessment findings. For example, if the pathomechanical diagnosis is that backward bending and side bending to the right exacerbate symptoms, then the prepositioning would include slight forward bending (tuck the chin) and side bending to the left. This position permits the gradual overload required to stimulate growth and the biochemical changes of consistent training.

The exercises are divided into mid pulls (Figs. 6–29 and 6–30), high pulls (Figs. 6–31 through 6–36), low pulls (Fig. 6–37), reciprocal push-pull (Fig. 6–38), and free weight exercises (Figs. 6–39 and 6–40). The pulling exercises are arranged and sequenced in this manner so that gradual

Text continued on page 221

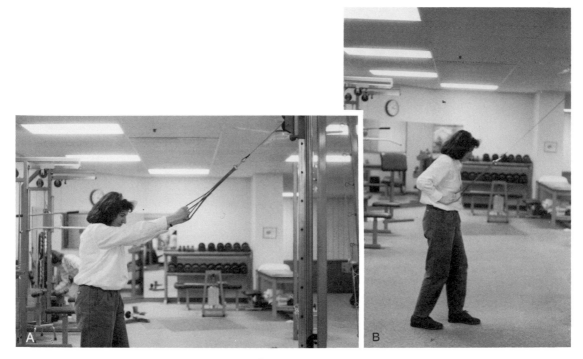

Figure 6–31. *(A)* Starting position for bilateral high pulls. Note position of head and neck and forward/back stance. *(B)* End position for bilateral high pulls. This exercise is in a midrange and safe for most upper-quarter problems.

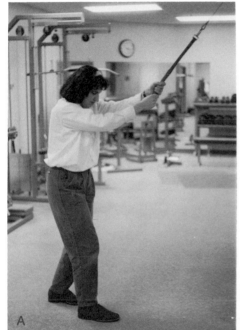
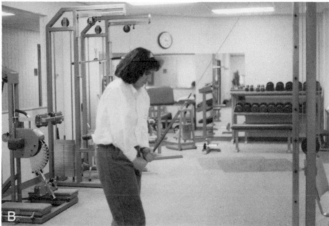

Figure 6–32. *(A)* Starting position for high central pulls. *(B)* End position for high central pulls. This exercise stroke is designed to initially exercise the posterior musculature of the mid and upper back. At the end of the stroke, the patient is instructed to slightly flex the trunk. This movement occurs by concentric contraction of the abdominal wall.

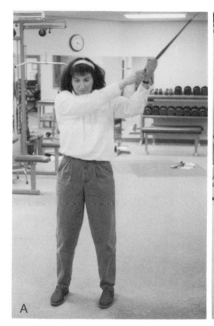
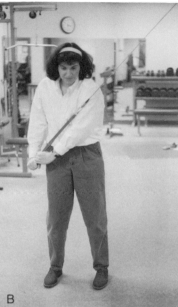

Figure 6–33. *(A)* Starting position for high diagonal pulls (stable trunk). *(B)* End position for high diagonal pulls (stable trunk). This exercise is designed to activate the oblique abdominal muscles as well as the anterior muscle of the left arm and the posterior muscles of the right arm.

Figure 6–34. *(A)* Starting position for high diagonal pulls (rotated trunk). *(B)* End position for high diagonal pulls (rotated trunk). The movement of the trunk in a forward bent and right rotated position further stimulates the musculature, progressing to a more functional motion. Diagonal pull should be done for each side.

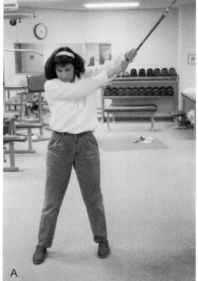
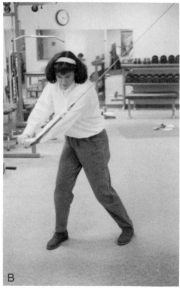

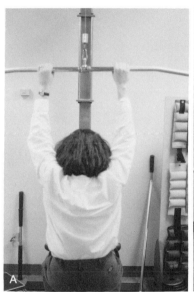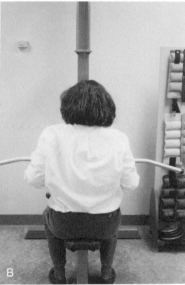

Figure 6–35. *(A)* Starting position for seated narrow gripped high pulls. *(B)* End position for seated narrow gripped high pulls (posterior view). The hand position can vary by pronating the forearms so that the hands are facing backward. This alteration permits a more natural movement and may be preferred. The position of the head must be maintained because returning to the starting position (eccentric contraction) tends to cause extension of the head and neck. Once the client is unable to sustain the desired position of the head and neck, the exercise should be terminated (reps to momentary fatigue or reps to substitution).

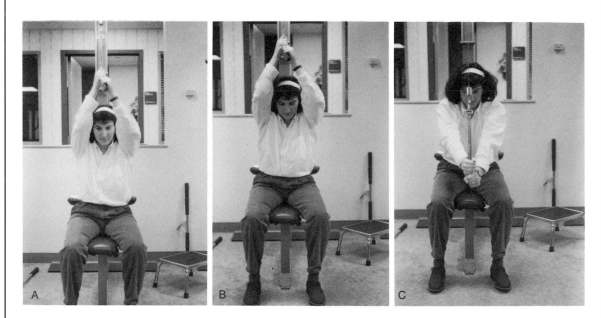

Figure 6–36. *(A)* Starting position for seated reverse central pulls. This exercise is excellent for the posterior upper arm, mid back, and abdominal wall. *(B)* Initial movement for seated reverse central pulls. The initial movement is slight trunk flexion. The instruction is to pull the anterior/inferior rib cage toward the top of the anterior pelvis (concentric rectus abdominous contraction). *(C)* End position (final stroke) for seated reverse central pulls. While maintaining the position of the rib cage, extend the humerus and elbows. The technique could be to do three or four reps of the final stroke and then return to the beginning position for the next repetition. The technique depends on clinician preference and which aspect of the exercise is to be emphasized.

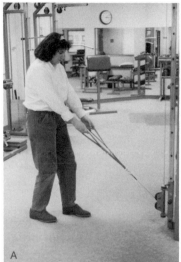 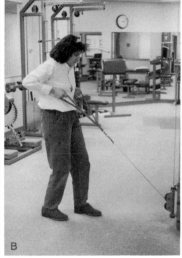 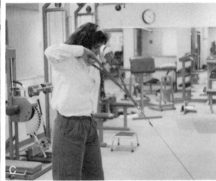

Figure 6–37. *(A)* Starting position for standing low pull. Note the position of the head, neck, and feet. It is not advised to stand with the feet parallel because of the resultant shear to the lumbar spine. *(B)* End position for standing low pull (mid stroke). The exercise should begin with a static stance but can progress to include a front-to-back weight shift—front on the downstroke and back on the upstroke. The trunk always is maintained on top of one foot. The motion stimulates dynamic contraction of other posterior muscles. *(C)* End position for standing low mid pull (high stroke). Varying the load and angle of pull is preferred during the training process. Continuation of a similar stoke until fatigue is preferred before altering the angle of pull. Once fatigue develops with the high stroke, the patient should be instructed to return to the original mid stroke for another set. This technique permits many reps of similar exercise before complete momentary fatigue. Low diagonal pulls can follow, which are similar to the techniques shown for the high pull position in Figures 6–33 and 6–34. Diagonal pull should be done for each side.

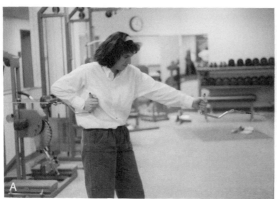
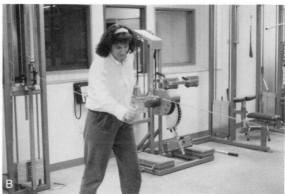

Figure 6–38. *(A)* Starting position for reciprocal push-pull. Standing between two pulleys, the patient is instructed to grasp a handle with each hand while standing facing one of the pulleys, as shown. *(B)* End position for reciprocal push-pull. This exercise is designed to create reciprocal contraction about the trunk and arms, which is an excellent way to train the oblique muscles of the abdominal wall. The patient is instructed to emphasize the motion of the rib cage. In this example, the right inferior anterior rib cage moves slightly toward the superior aspect of the left ilium (concentric contraction of the right external oblique and left internal oblique).

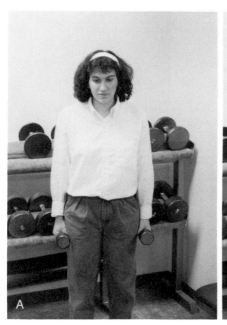
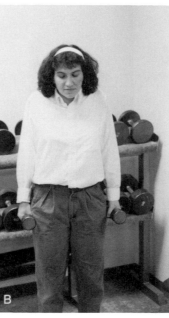

Figure 6–39. *(A)* Starting position for standing shoulder shrugs. Because this exercise results specifically in compression forces directed to the cervical spine, the head and neck position should be emphasized. Note the tucked, slightly flexed neck and tucked chin. *(B)* End position for standing shoulder shrugs. Once this exercise is completed, the angle can be changed by bending slightly forward at the waist. This change in position focuses the forces of the exercise to other aspects of the scapular elevators and retractors. Before instructing the patient as to this change of position, the clinician should make sure that there is no problem with the tissues of the low back.

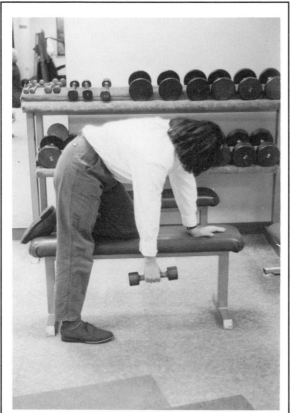

Figure 6–40. (A) Starting position for one-arm row. Note the stability of this exercise; all body parts are stabilized and the motion is concentrated only at the right upper quarter in this example. The action of the exercise is flexing the right elbow, extending the humerus, and retracting the scapula. The repetitions should be performed until either the weight-bearing arm or shoulder becomes fatigued or quality range of motion cannot be completed. This is an excellent way to strengthen the muscles of the upper quarter, and it is a variation of the previously described pulling exercise.

progression of forces can be introduced into the upper quarter. The mid pull is the least stressful for the head and neck, and the low pull is the most stressful. It is not necessary to have equipment to perform the pulling exercises; they can be carried out with resistance tubing.

The exercises shown in Figures 6–29 through 6–40 are an example of an upper-quarter training routine that can vary, depending on equip-

ment available and the details of the patient's clinical picture. The patient realizes the positive changes intrinsic to the training process if a program can be individually tailored for the patient and the condition and is consistently performed for 4 to 6 weeks.[5, 7]

Objective No. 4: Biomechanical Counseling

Biomechanical counseling refers to assisting the patient in establishing the intensity, frequency, and duration of loads imparted to the upper quarter and in minimizing destructive movement patterns that exacerbate the symptom. It is also an important part of the patient education process, as previously mentioned, to assist the patient in integrating the many aspects of the syndrome that, when coupled together, exacerbate the symptom. Specific short- and long-term goals should be established. The clinician's ability to set and meet realistic short-term goals is the key to the successful management of these conditions. The patient begins to gain confidence in the clinician as short-term goals are realized, and it is important, especially in the initial part of treatment, that the clinician communicate with the patient regarding the expected outcome of the treatment plan.

Other areas that should be emphasized during the biomechanical counseling for the patient with upper-quarter dysfunction include sleeping postures and use of the proper pillow. The patient should be counseled to position the head so that it remains in a midrange position throughout the night. Unless the head and shoulders have to be propped up to aid in breathing, the patient with neck complaints should use a pillow that is supportive and places the head and neck in a neutral position. There are many specific designs for cervical pillows that may or may not be advantageous, depending on the patient's positional needs. These needs are determined during the assessment process that identifies what positions and forces reproduce the familiar symptoms.

The patient whose symptoms are exacerbated by backward bending and who wears bifocals should be made aware of the similarities of the positions. Prolonged positions used when reading should be examined as to the forces that are generated into and through the spine. These are a few examples of what might be discussed with a patient so that he or she can begin to relate all activities to decreasing unwanted forces to the cervical spine. Self-management means the analysis of all activities of daily living as they relate to the syndrome.

Other activities that may exacerbate the symptoms of a patient with upper-quarter syndrome are excessive overhead work such as painting or carpentry, prolonged positions that may exacerbate neural tension signs if recognized during the assessment, and repetitive lifting without proper stabilization of the head and shoulders.

SUMMARY

This text has attempted to develop a pragmatic approach toward the assessment and treatment of mechanical neck pain based on the understanding of neuromusculoskeletal science. Correlating the assessment findings to appropriate decision-making during the treatment process is the primary focus. In order to provide a more standardized approach to treatment, four objectives have been described under which most treatment techniques can be placed.

To ensure successful outcomes from the treatment plan, the clinician must develop a relationship with the patient based on common goals of improving function and education for self-management. Health care professionals must remain cognizant of the importance of effectively directing the responsibility of control to the patient by way of education, which allows the clinician to then serve as a teacher of the healing and exercise processes, and a facilitator to an active, healthy life-style.

REFERENCES

1. Drugs used for spasticity and muscle spasm. *In* Neurologic Drugs. AMA (Drug Evaluation Subscription, Division of Toxicology) 4:1–17, 1991.
2. Evjenth O, Hamberg J: The spinal column and the TM joint. *In* Muscle Stretching in Manual Therapy, a Clinical Manual. Vol 2. Sweden, Alfta Rehab, 1980, pp 26–86.
3. Kaltenborn FM: The Spine: Basic Evaluation and Mobilization Techniques. Norway, Olaf Norlis Bokhandel; USA Distrib. OPTP, P.O. Box 47009, Minneapolis, MN 55447-0009, 1993.
4. Kellet J: Acute soft tissue injuries—a review of the literature. Med Sci Sports Exerc 18:5, 489–500, 1986.
5. Komi PV: Training of muscle strength and power: Interaction of neuromotoric, hypertrophic and mechanical factors. Int J Sports Med 7[Suppl]:10–15, 1986.
6. Maitland GD: Vertebral Manipulation. London, Butterworths, 1973.
7. Sale DG, MacDougall JD, Upton ARM, McComas AJ: Effect of strength training upon motoneuron excitability in man. Med Sci Sports Exerc 15:57–62, 1983.
8. van der Muelen JCH: Present state of knowledge on processes of healing in collagen structures. Int J Sports Med 3:4–8, 1982.
9. Waddell G: A new clinical model for the treatment of low-back pain. Spine 12:632–644, 1987.
10. Waddell G, Main CJ, Morris EW, et al: Chronic low back pain, psychological distress and illness behavior. Spine 9:209–213, 1984.
11. Wolf CJ: Generation of acute pain: Central mechanisms. Br Med Bull 47:3, 523–533, 1991.
12. Woo SL-Y, Buckwalter JA: Injury and Repair of the Musculoskeletal Soft Tissues. Park Ridge, Illinois, American Academy of Orthopedic Surgeons, 1988.

INDEX

223

ISBN 0-7216-6640-X

90071

9 780721 666402